Fundamentals of Intravitreal Injections

A Guide for Ophthalmic Nurse Practitioners and Allied Health Professionals

Fundamentals of Intravitreal Injections

A Guide for Ophthalmic Nurse Practitioners and Allied Health Professionals

Mr Salman Waqar
FRCOphth
Consultant Ophthalmologist
Royal Eye Infirmary
Plymouth
United Kingdom

Mr Jonathan C. Park
FRCOphth
Consultant Ophthalmologist
Musgrove Park Hospital
Taunton
United Kingdom

World Scientific

NEW JERSEY • LONDON • SINGAPORE • BEIJING • SHANGHAI • HONG KONG • TAIPEI • CHENNAI • TOKYO

Published by

World Scientific Publishing Co. Pte. Ltd.

5 Toh Tuck Link, Singapore 596224

USA office: 27 Warren Street, Suite 401-402, Hackensack, NJ 07601

UK office: 57 Shelton Street, Covent Garden, London WC2H 9HE

Library of Congress Cataloging-in-Publication Data

Names: Waqar, Salman, 1970– author. | Park, Jonathan C., author.
Title: Fundamentals of intravitreal injections : a guide for ophthalmic nurse practitioners and allied health professionals / Salman Waqar, Jonathan C. Park.
Description: New Jersey : World Scientific, 2018. | Includes index.
Identifiers: LCCN 2018014810| ISBN 9789813239784 (hardcover : alk. paper) | ISBN 9813239786 (hardcover : alk. paper)
Subjects: | MESH: Eye Diseases--therapy | Intravitreal Injections--methods | Eye Diseases--nursing | Intravitreal Injections--nursing | Handbooks
Classification: LCC RE88 | NLM WW 39 | DDC 617.7/0231--dc23
LC record available at https://lccn.loc.gov/2018014810

British Library Cataloguing-in-Publication Data

A catalogue record for this book is available from the British Library.

First published 2018 (Hardcover)
Reprinted 2020 (in paperback edition)
ISBN 978-981-122-132-3 (pbk)

For any available supplementary material, please visit
http://www.worldscientific.com/worldscibooks/10.1142/10977#t=suppl

CONTENTS

ABOUT THE AUTHORS

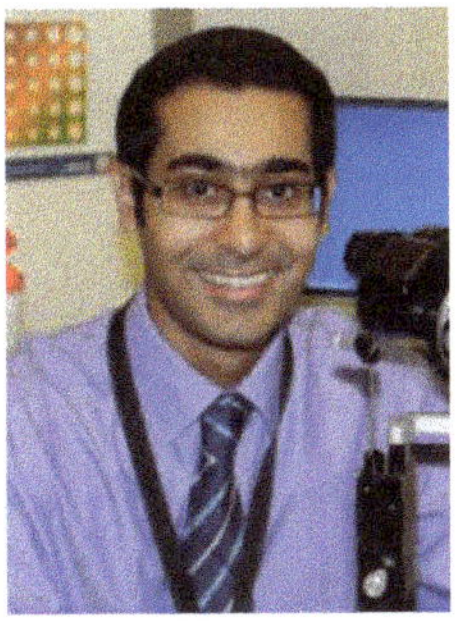

Salman Waqar completed his medical degree at the University of Health Sciences, Pakistan. He undertook basic training in general surgery (Sheffield), followed by specialist ophthalmology training in the beautiful south-west of England. He has published extensively on the use of virtual reality training systems in ophthalmology and has also designed various innovative instruments to enhance patient safety. He is regularly involved with training ophthalmic nurse practitioners and is an instructor for the course on "Basic Microsurgical Skills" at the Royal College of Ophthalmologists. His prior foray into the world of books included contributing to one related to ophthalmology training (refraction and retinoscopy), a science fiction novel and a children's book. Outside of work he is an enthusiastic triathlete and squash player. You can find out more about him on www.salmanwaqar.net.

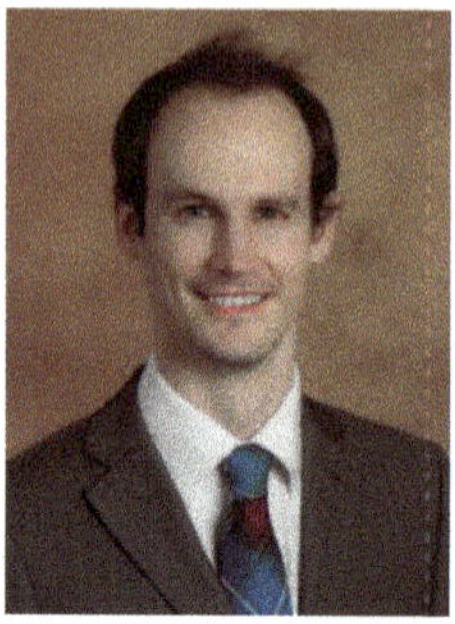

Jonathan Park qualified as a doctor from the University of Bristol in 2005, which included an additional year of research in anatomical sciences. He completed his training in South West England, followed by an internationally respected retinal specialist fellowship at the University of Toronto, Canada. Since 2015 he has worked as a Consultant Ophthalmic Surgeon with a specialist interest in surgical and medical retina, based at Musgrove Park Hospital, Taunton. His research publications relate to infections after eye surgery, intravitreal injection and virtual reality eye surgery. He has been conferred with national and international research awards, and has served as an invited speaker on research at the Royal College of Ophthalmologists Annual Congress. He enjoys endurance cycling and surfing, and is beginning to understand the art of craft cider production.

FOREWORD

I am delighted to write a Foreword for this book, which addresses the need to provide a detailed and clear account of how nurse practitioners and allied health professionals should be trained to perform intravitreal injections in a controlled environment with patient safety being paramount.

This book uses a step-by-step approach, starting with the basic anatomy and building up to the technique itself, whilst emphasising the awareness and management of complications. It also offers detailed guidance on how eye units should formally train practitioners in this technique, and ensure that all clinical governance issues about maintaining patient safety are addressed.

There is an ever-increasing demand for eye unit resources to provide intravitreal injections for treatment of wet macular degeneration, centre-involved diabetic maculopathy and vein occlusions. A well-trained practitioner can provide not only excellent technical expertise but also continuity of care for such patients, who usually require regular injections. The Royal College of Ophthalmologists and the Macular Society support the use of nurse practitioners and allied health professionals for intravitreal injections, and the authors are to be congratulated on presenting a timely and well-written wealth of information that will also be useful for ophthalmologists in training.

Peter Simcock
FRCP, FRCS, FRCOphth
Consultant Ophthalmologist
West of England Eye Unit, Exeter
October 2017

ACKNOWLEDGEMENTS

We are indebted to our lovely patient for her permission to photograph the procedure; to Sue Ashton (Ophthalmic Nurse Practitioner, Royal Eye Infirmary, Plymouth), who performed the injection; and to Khadijah Azhar for her beautiful illustrations. Our gratitude also goes to Mr Roger Gray and Mr Edward Herbert (Consultant Ophthalmologists, Musgrove Park Hospital, Taunton), for providing the excellent fundus fluorescein angiography (FFA) images.

1

INTRODUCTION

Age-related macular degeneration is the commonest cause of visual impairment registration in the UK. Intravitreal injections (injections into the vitreous gel of the eye) of antivascular endothelial growth factors (anti-VEGF's) such as Lucentis® (ranibizumab), Avastin® (bevacizumab) and Eylea® (aflibercept) are now widely accepted to reduce the progression of "wet" macular degeneration. There is also good evidence of their efficacy in macular oedema secondary to diabetes and vein occlusions.

Ophthalmic nurse practitioners and allied health professionals are increasingly becoming invaluable team members for delivering intravitreal injections, particularly as the clinical demand grows. We have written this handbook to aid our colleagues in such an endeavour and hope that it will provide concise, relevant information in a format that is easy to carry around and access. Towards the end we have outlined our experience in designing a training structure and it is our sincere hope that this will provide a framework for others too. We have extensive experience in organising wetlab sessions for both ophthalmic trainees and nurse practitioners, and have added some easy tips for readers to set up a session of their own. The appendices contain the latest information on basic life support and anaphylaxis treatment. Whilst the practitioner will always be in a well-supported environment and emergency response teams will be just a phone call away, it is beneficial to be familiar with these algorithms. The book is aimed primarily at nurse practitioners and allied health professionals, but we are confident that it will also be a useful reference for junior ophthalmic trainees learning how to perform intravitreal injections.

We wish you all the best for your career as part of the retinal team!

Salman Waqar
Jonathan Park

2

BASICS

In order to be proficient in intravitreal injections, it is crucial to appreciate the structure of the eye and how this knowledge can be used to give a safe injection.

The eye is a highly specialised organ of photoreception. This is a process by which light energy from the environment produces changes in specialised nerve cells in the retina (rods and cones). These changes result in action potentials (the electrical voltage across a cell) that are subsequently relayed to the optic nerve and then to the brain, where the information is processed and consciously appreciated as vision.

The eye is an approximate sphere 2.5 cm in diameter (equivalent to an axial length of 25 mm), with a volume of 5 mL (fills 1/6 of the orbit, whose volume is 30 mL). It consists of three basic layers.

THE THREE LAYERS OF THE EYE

1. **The fibrous corneoscleral coat** consists of the cornea and the sclera.

- **The Cornea**

This is the anteriormost, transparent window of the eye. The cornea meets the sclera at the limbus, which is also where

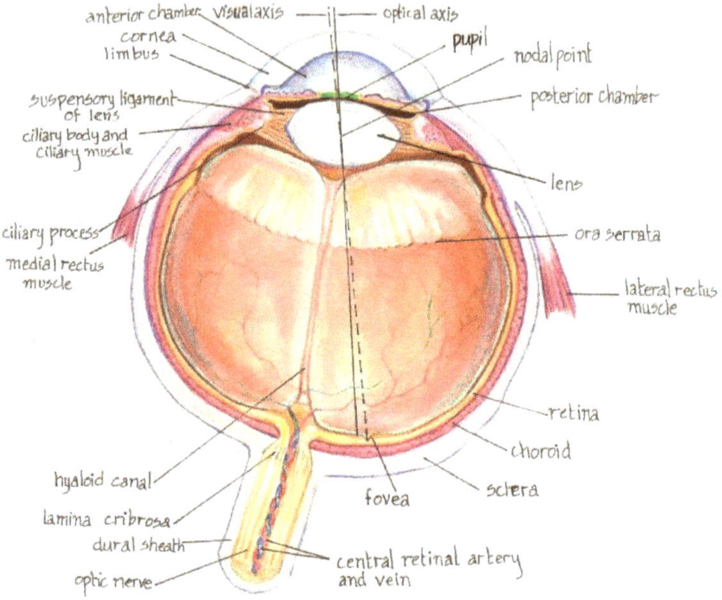

Fig. 2.1. The eye in cross section.

the conjunctiva ends. The conjunctiva covers the sclera but not the cornea. The cornea is kept transparent by its avascularity and the innermost monolayer of cells (endothelium), which pumps fluid out of the corneal stroma. It presents a tough barrier to trauma and infection, and is responsible for about 2/3 of the eyes' refractive power (the remaining 1/3 comes from the lens).

- **The Sclera**

This is an opaque white fibrous coat that also protects the eye and maintains its shape owing to inherent structural integrity.

2. **The uvea (or uveal tract)** is the middle vascular pigmented layer of the eye and consists of the iris, ciliary body and choroid.

- **The Iris**

This is a thin contractile circular disc, analogous to the diaphragm of a camera. The iris separates the anterior and posterior chambers, which are filled with aqueous humour and are in continuity through an opening, the pupil. The iris is attached by its root at the "angle" (iridocorneal) of the anterior chamber where it merges with the ciliary body and trabecular meshwork. Aqueous humour drains mainly through the trabecular meshwork, which is visible using a mirror within a contact lens called a gonioscope.

- **The Ciliary Body**

  This is approximately 6 mm in width and is responsible for the production of aqueous humour. It also contains muscles, which are attached to the zonular ligaments of the lens (changing its shape on contraction to focus or accommodate). It has two parts: the pars plicata and the pars plana. The pars plicata is the anterior part. It is 2 mm long (measured from the limbus) and contains about 70 ciliary processes which are the site of attachment for the aforementioned zonular ligaments The pars plana is a posterior flat area 4 mm long. As the sclera and cornea are relatively rigid, excess production or reduced drainage of aqueous humour or injection of substances into the eye leads to raised intraocular pressure (normally this is up to 21 mmHg). Intraocular pressure is high immediately after intravitreal injections (it can be as high as 60 mmHg). Normalisation of the pressure usually occurs over 30 min after injection and is dependent on aqueous humour outflow through the trabecular meshwork. The safest site for administering intravitreal injections is through the pars plana. This is because it lies behind the lens and in front of the retina, thus avoiding damage to either of these structures.

- **The Choroid**

  This highly pigmented and vascular posterior portion lies between the sclera and the retina, and extends forwards to the ciliary body. Its principal function is to nourish the outer layers of the retina and prevent unwanted light from reflecting back through the retina. It is composed of an outer layer of large-calibre blood vessels, which divide into smaller-diameter vessels and ultimately form the choriocapillaris (a network of capillaries). These drain into the vortex veins, which ultimately drain into the superior and inferior ophthalmic veins. The innermost layer of the choroid is a membrane called Bruch's membrane. The basal portion of the retinal pigment epithelium is attached to this membrane. This is of clinical importance, as in age-related macular degeneration it is Bruch's membrane that is breached by abnormal choroidal blood vessels, leading to pathognomic features of the disease (as will be discussed later, in the imaging section).

3. **The retina (neural layer)** is where photoreception occurs. It consists of two primary layers: the inner neurosensory retina and an outer layer called the retinal pigment epithelium (RPE). Anatomically it comprises the following regions:

- **The macula** (Latin for "patch"; same as the macula lutea) is the area within the main vascular arcades and is 5–6 mm in diameter. Cone photoreceptors are mostly concentrated here for fine resolution (maximum density in the fovea).
- **The fovea** (Latin for "pit") is the central 1.5-mm-diameter area of the macula. The foveola is the central 0.35-mm-diameter area of the fovea (Fig. 2.2).
- **The optic disc** is 1.5 mm in diameter. It contains no normal retinal layers or photoreceptors (thus causing the blind spot) and is the area where nerve fibres of retinal ganglion cells pierce the sclera to enter the optic nerve. The central pale thinned area of the disc forms the cup, which becomes progressively enlarged through loss of ganglion cells in glaucoma. The cup's vertical diameter is measured in relation to the disc's diameter when one is monitoring a patient with glaucoma (referred to as the cup-to-disc ratio).
- **The peripheral retina** is rich in rod photoreceptors which provide acuity at low levels of illumination.
- **The ora serrata** is where the peripheral retina ends. This is approximately 7 mm from the limbus.

The Retina in Cross Section

The retina consists of 10 layers. From posterior to anterior these are (Fig. 2.3):

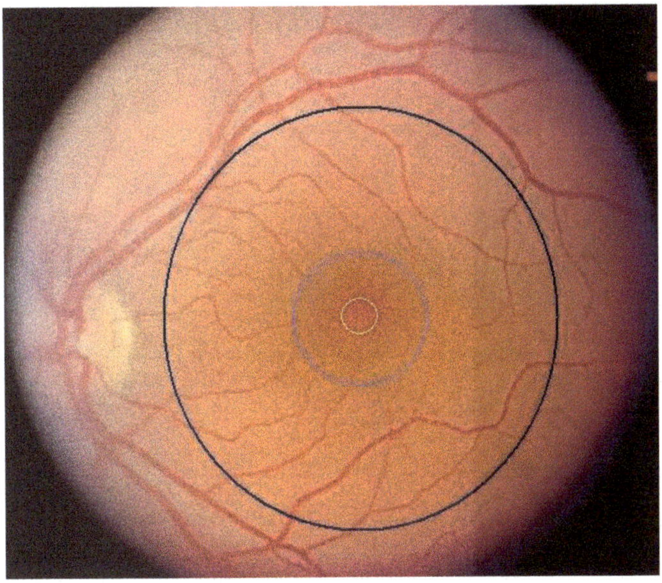

Fig. 2.2. A normal fundus photograph (left eye) showing the approximate locations of the macula (black circle), fovea (blue circle) and foveola (yellow circle).

1. **Retinal pigment epithelium (RPE).** This is a monolayer of cells which have several functions, including maintaining the adhesion of the neurosensory retina, rendering the subretinal space dry, removing shed portions of photoreceptor outer segments, contributing to the transport and storage of metabolites/vitamins and providing a blood retinal permeability barrier.
2. **Photoreceptor layer.** This contains rod and cone inner/outer segments. The outer segments contain the visual pigments that are responsible for absorption of light and initiation of the neuroelectrical impulse, whilst the inner segments contain the cellular apparatus required to provide energy, e.g. mitochondria. The junction of the two segments is visible on high resolution OCT, as discussed later.
3. **External limiting membrane.** This is a histological feature of the retina. It is a dark line caused by junctions between

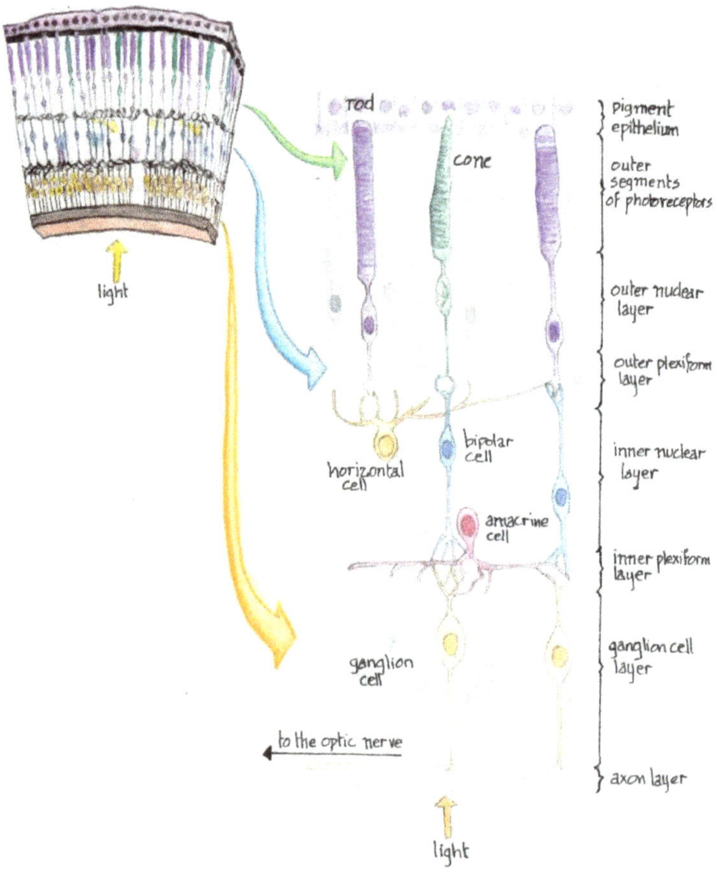

Fig. 2.3. The retina in cross section.

photoreceptors and Müller cells. It is located between the photoreceptor and outer nuclear layers.

4. **Outer nuclear layer.** This contains the nucleated cell bodies of the rods and cones. Cones subserve fine resolution essential for reading, spatial resolution and colour vision, whilst rods sense contrast, brightness and motion. Rods are also mainly responsible for peripheral and night vision.
5. **Outer plexiform layer.** This contains the cone and rod axons. It also contains dendrites of horizontal and bipolar cells.

6. **Inner nuclear layer.** This contains the nuclei of horizontal cells, bipolar cells, amacrine cells and Müller cells.
7. **Inner plexiform layer.** This contains the axons of bipolar cells and amacrine cells along with dendrites of ganglion cells.
8. **Ganglion cell layer.** This contains the nuclei of ganglion cells.
9. **Nerve fibre layer (axon layer).** This is formed by the axons of ganglion cells traversing the retina to leave the eye at the optic disc.
10. **Inner limiting membrane.** This is a membrane on the inner surface of the retina.

THE VITREOUS

The vitreous is a thick transparent substance that fills the centre of the eye between the lens and the retina. It is composed mainly of water and constitutes about 2/3 of the eye's volume. The viscous properties of the vitreous allow the eye to return to its normal shape if compressed.

In children, the vitreous has a consistency similar to that of an egg white. With age it gradually thins and becomes more liquid. The vitreous is firmly attached to certain areas of the retina. As it thins, it separates from the retina, often causing floaters. This may ultimately lead to separation from areas around the optic disc and retinal periphery (a condition called posterior vitreous detachment, or PVD). There are various causes of retinal detachment (detachment of the neurosensory retina from the RPE), but the commonest cause is due to pulling forces on the peripheral retina by the posterior lining of the vitreous at the time of a PVD. Fortunately, most PVD's do not result in retinal detachment, since although PVD is common, retinal detachment is relatively rare. PVD itself is not sight-threatening but, if it is associated with a retinal detachment, treatment is typically required to prevent loss of sight. During intravitreal injections, incorrect placement of the needle through the retina can cause a tear and lead to a retinal detachment too.

THE LENS

In addition to appreciating the three layers of the eye, knowledge of the lens is important in order to avoid inadvertent damage.

The lens is a highly organised system of specialised cells within a transparent capsule. Situated in the anterior segment of the eye, it provides a third of the refractive power of the eye. Zonules from the ciliary body hold the lens in place.

A cataract (Latin for "waterfall") is regarded as a visually significant opaqueness of the lens for which age is the commonest risk factor. Cataract surgery is the commonest operation performed in the UK. Damage by a needle during an intravitreal injection can lead to rapid cataract development and problems due to sudden swelling of the lens.

3

INVESTIGATIONS

Every patient presenting for an intravitreal injection will have gone through an investigative process in the clinic. The ophthalmic nurse practitioner will inevitably come across the results of these patients either in the clinic or whilst looking through the notes prior to injection. Also, nurse practitioners are now increasingly reviewing patients in clinics and may in the future be an integral part of "virtual" clinics where they will carry out investigations at a peripheral site and the clinician will review the results in the hospital. Therefore, an understanding of the basic investigative techniques employed is beneficial. Here we discuss the essentials of optical coherence tomography and fundus fluorescein angiography, alongside an introduction to new modalities such as optical coherence tomography angiography and ultra-widefield fundus imaging.

OPTICAL COHERENCE TOMOGRAPHY (OCT)

OCT allows high-resolution cross-sectional (tomographic) images of the retina to be obtained in a non-invasive manner. It works by measuring the properties of light waves reflected from tissue (similar to sound wave measurements in ultrasonography). However, the utilisation of light instead of sound

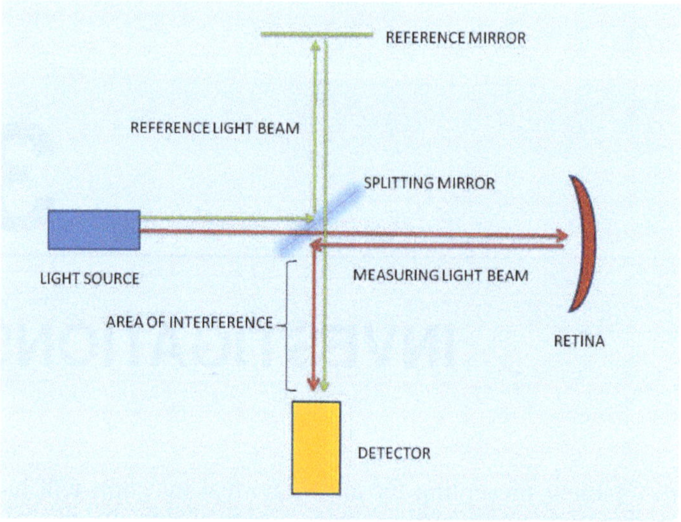

Fig. 3.1. Schematic diagram of a Michelson interferometer demonstrating the principle of optical coherence tomography.

presents a technical challenge. The speed of light makes direct measurements on the reflected waves impossible. In OCT systems, this hurdle is overcome through the use of a technique called interferometry. In interferometry, a beam of light is divided into a measuring beam and a reference beam. The reconvergence of light reflected from the tissue of interest and light reflected from a reference path produces characteristic patterns of interference that are dependent on the mismatch between the reflected waves (Fig. 3.1). Because the time delay and amplitude of one of the waves (i.e. the reference path) are known, the time delay and intensity of light returning from the sample tissue may then be extracted from the interference pattern. A two-dimensional or three-dimensional image of the retina is then created in which "hot" colours denote stronger reflectivity and "cool" colours weaker reflectivity. Thus, highly reflective tissue is reddish-white, whereas less reflective tissue is bluish-black. Alternatively, the OCT image can be displayed on a grey scale, where more highly reflected light is brighter than less highly reflected light.

The first hyper-reflective layer detected is the internal limiting membrane (ILM). The retinal nerve fibre layer and both the inner and outer plexiform layers are seen as hyper-reflective. The ganglion cell layer and both the inner and outer nuclear layers are hypo-reflective. Within the photoreceptor layer the external limiting membrane and the ellipsoid zones (sometimes still called the inner/outer segment junction) appear hyper-reflective. The ellipsoid zone is an important area, since if damaged it often correlates with poor visual function. The RPE appears hyper-reflective too (Fig. 3.2).

There are two types of OCT scan machines:

1. *Time domain OCT*. This is the older generation of OCT scan machines. Here interference patterns are assessed as a function of time, and therefore the resolution is low and it takes

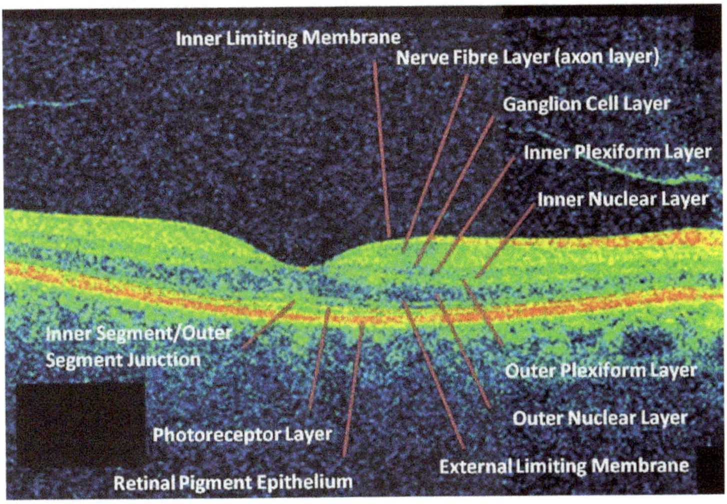

Fig. 3.2. A normal spectral domain OCT showing an approximate correlation of the anatomical layers. Notice the higher resolution as compared to time domain systems.

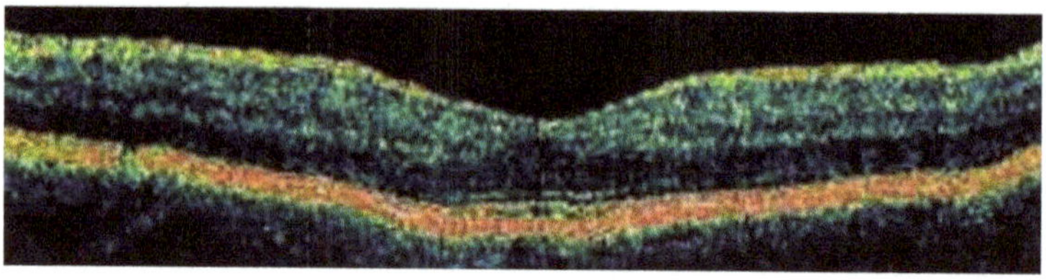

Fig. 3.3. A time domain OCT of a normal macula.

longer to acquire an image (able to visualise structures down to 10 micrometres and acquire images at a rate of 400 scans per second); see Fig. 3.3.

2. *Spectral domain OCT*. These newer generation systems use spectral interferometry and a mathematical function called Fourier transformation to assess interference patterns as a function of frequency rather than time. This allows light scattered from different depths within the tissue to be measured simultaneously. In simple terms, images can be acquired more quickly than in time domain systems (over 20,000 scans per second) and the resolution is higher (able to visualise structures down to 3 micrometres).

Common pathological appearances seen on an OCT scan are:

1. Choroidal neovascularisation (CNV) or "wet" age-related macular degeneration (AMD) is caused by abnormal choroidal blood vessels breaking through the RPE. An OCT scan will display an RPE disturbance, as well as subretinal and intraretinal fluid, as shown in Fig. 3.4.
2. A pigment epithelial detachment (PED) can be seen in both "dry" and "wet" AMD. In the "dry" instance, deposition of abnormal degenerative material (drusen) between the RPE and Bruch's membrane causes the RPE to detach, resulting in a dome-shaped elevation, as shown in Fig. 3.5. This is called a serous PED. A PED can also be seen in a form of wet

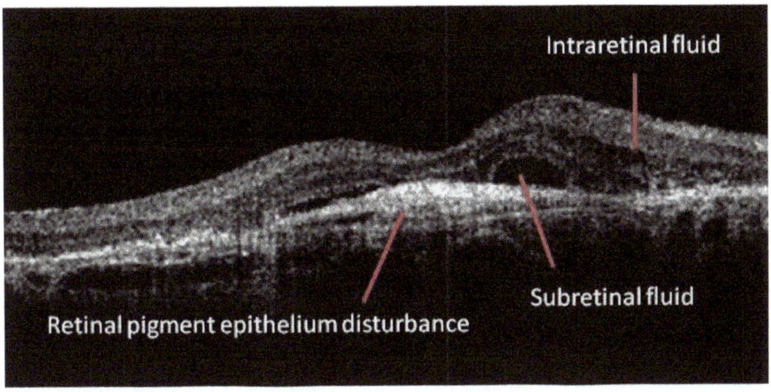

Fig. 3.4. A spectral domain OCT of an eye with "wet" age-related macular degeneration (choroidal neovascularisation), showing intraretinal fluid, subretinal fluid and RPE disturbance.

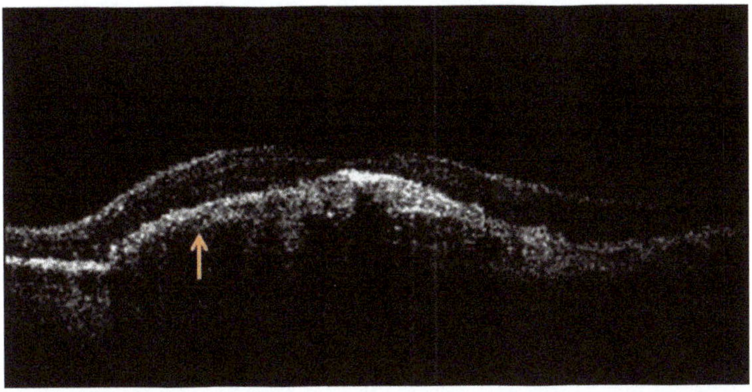

Fig. 3.5. An OCT showing a PED (arrow). Note the dome-shaped elevation of the retinal pigment epithelium.

AMD (called occult CNV) where abnormal choroidal blood vessels are present between Bruch's membrane and the RPE, again causing the RPE to detach. This is called a fibrovascular PED. It is not possible to differentiate between the two kinds of PED's based on OCT alone. A combination of fundoscopy, OCT and fluorescein angiography can help reach a diagnosis.

3. Cystoid macular oedema can be seen in eyes with inflammation (uveitis) or following a vein occlusion. This presents as cystic spaces within the retina, as shown in Fig. 3.6.
4. Diabetic macular oedema presents simply as intraretinal fluid (Fig. 3.7).

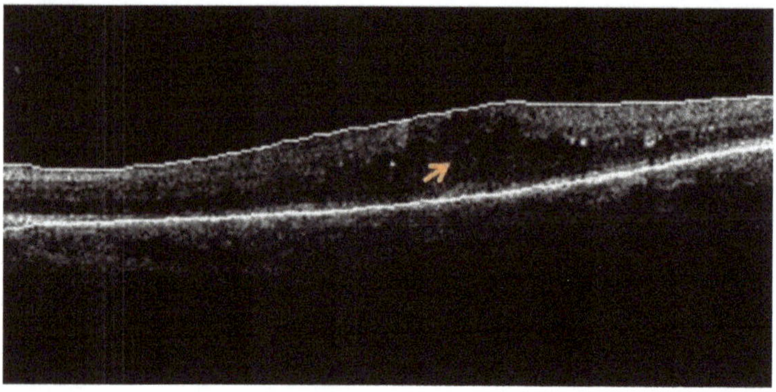

Fig. 3.6. An OCT showing cystic intraretinal spaces consistent with cystoid macular oedema (arrow).

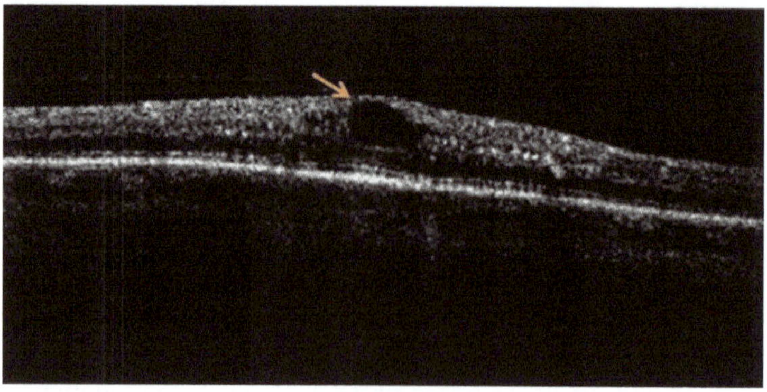

Fig. 3.7. An OCT of a diabetic patient, showing intraretinal fluid (arrow) indicative of diabetic macular oedema.

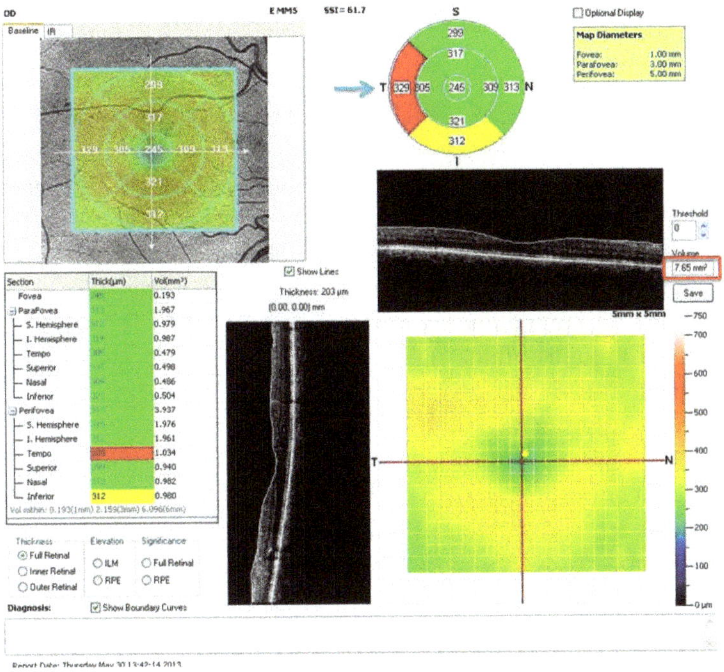

Fig. 3.8. A full-page report of a normal OCT (right eye). Such reports provide various other useful parameters for serial monitoring, in addition to a retinal cross section. Macular volume (red box) and numerical values of macular thickness (blue arrow) are particularly useful.

Further reading

Further information on the science of OCT scans can be gained from these articles which we have referenced:

1. Jaffe GJ, Caprioli J (2004). Optical coherence tomography to detect and manage retinal disease and glaucoma. *Am J Ophthalmol* **137**(1): 156–169.
2. Keane PA, Patel PJ, Liakopoulos S, *et al.* (2012). Evaluation of age-related macular degeneration with optical coherence tomography. *Surv Ophthalmol* **57**(5): 389–414.

FUNDUS FLUORESCEIN ANGIOGRAPHY (FFA)

This technique involves intravenously injecting a dye (fluorescein sodium) to allow visualisation of the retinal and choroidal circulation alongside any associated abnormalities. Fluorescence is the property of certain substances to emit a light of longer wavelength when stimulated by light of a lower wavelength. Fluorescein sodium is excited by blue light (490 nm) and emits yellow–green light (530 nm). It is water-soluble and once within the circulation approximately 80% of it is bound to plasma proteins whilst the rest remains unbound. Its passage through the retinal and choroidal circulation follows certain anatomical principles:

- The choriocapillaris (the smallest blood vessels in the choroid) are permeable to the unbound fluorescein. This leaks out and passes through Bruch's membrane but cannot pass through the retinal pigment epithelium. Tight junctions here prevent any further passage and this forms the "outer blood–retinal barrier."
- The retinal blood vessels also have tight junctions that prevent any fluorescein (both bound and unbound) from passing out. This is called the "inner blood–retinal barrier."

Usually, 5 mL of 10% fluorescein sodium is injected as a bolus intravenously. A cobalt blue excitation filter attached to the camera allows only blue light to reach the retina. The fluorescein is excited and only yellow–green light is allowed back to the camera via a yellow–green barrier filter. A wide-gauge cannula should ideally be inserted, as this will be invaluable for management should treatment be needed for anaphylaxis. A red-free image is usually taken prior to injecting fluorescein. This is done with a yellow–green filter in place, thus blocking red light. As a result red structures appear black, allowing better visualisation of any vascular abnormalities. Localised retinal structural abnormalities can also become more evident (Fig. 3.9).

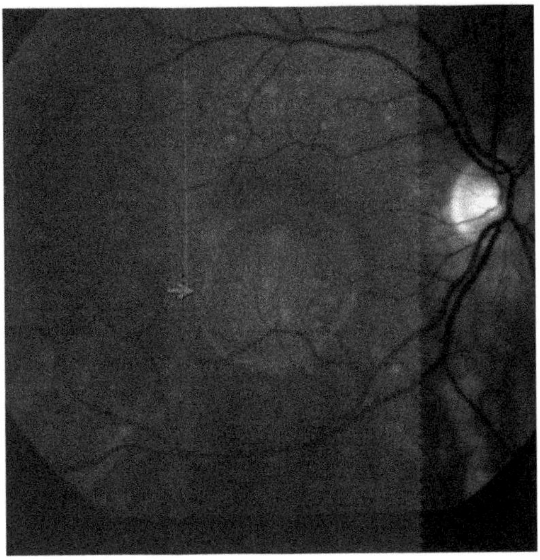

Fig. 3.9. Red-free image. A localised retinal disturbance can be seen (arrow).

A normal FFA demonstrates the following well-recognised phases:

1. *Pre-arterial or choroidal phase.* It takes approximately 10–15 sec for the fluorescein to reach the eye following injection. This can be longer in patients with systemic disorders causing circulatory insufficiency, e.g. atherosclerosis. Once in the eye, the fluorescein enters the choroidal circulation a second earlier than the retinal circulation. Thus, the first phase presents a diffuse leakage of dye from the choriocapillaris, known as a "choroidal flush." The choroid appears fluorescent but there is no dye yet in the retinal vessels.
2. *Arterial phase.* As the name implies, this phase shows the retinal arteries filling up with dye a second or so after the choroidal phase (Fig. 3.10).
3. *Arteriovenous phase.* In this phase the veins begin to show laminar flow (Fig. 3.11). This means that the dye is flowing

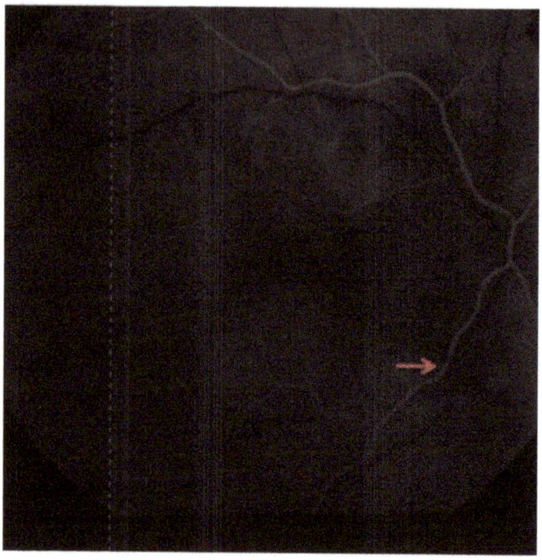

Fig. 3.10. An FFA showing arterial filling with fluorescein sodium dye (arrow).

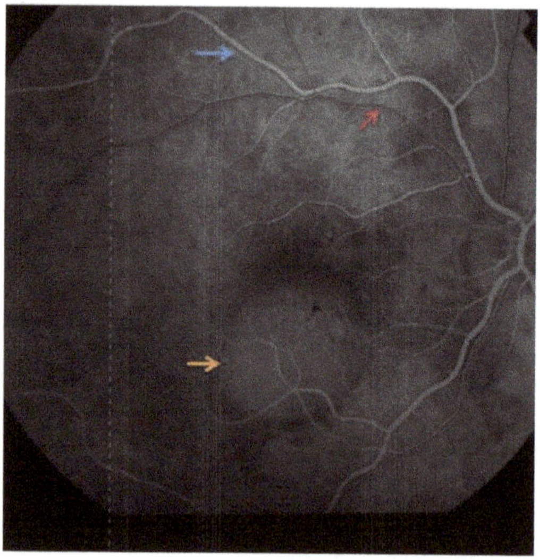

Fig. 3.11. An FFA showing arteries filled up (blue arrow) with laminar venous flow (red arrow). Note the localised dye pooling (orange arrow) indicating a pigment epithelial detachment. This is a pathological finding and would not be expected in a normal FFA.

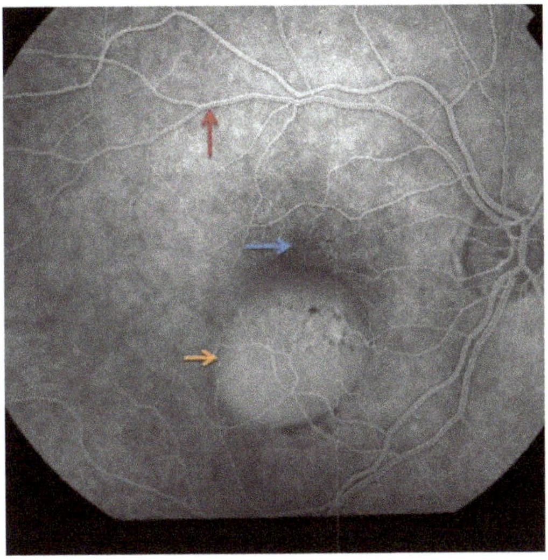

Fig. 3.12. The venous phase, showing complete venous filling (red arrow). The fovea is dark (blue arrow). A localised subretinal pooling of dye (orange arrow) indicates a pigment epithelial detachment. This is a pathological finding and would not be expected in a normal FFA.

adjacent to the venous walls initially due to faster plasma flow adjacent to the vessel wall.

4. *Venous phase*. During this phase the veins fill up completely with fluorescein (Fig. 3.12). The fovea remains dark, owing to:

   - absent blood vessels (this is also called the foveal avascular zone);
   - high density of the pigment xanthophyll blocking the background choroidal fluorescence;
   - larger RPE cells with higher concentrations of the pigments melanin and lipofuscin blocking the background choroidal fluorescence.

By now around 30 sec have elapsed since the dye injection and its first pass through the eye is complete.

5. *Late phase*. This is also called the recirculation phase. Here the dye continuously recirculates through the eye, the fluorescence getting less intense as time passes until complete absence by around 10 min. The optic disc continues to show staining for a while afterwards. Sometimes the preceding four phases are collectively referred to as the early phase.

   FFA's are interpreted in terms of areas of increased and decreased fluorescence. These are called "hyperfluorescent" and "hypofluorescent" respectively. Whilst looking at an FFA image one can tell which eye the image is from by ascertaining which side the optic disc is on, i.e. if the optic disc is on the right side of the image, then we are looking at an FFA of the right eye, and vice versa. Areas of hyperfluorescence are seen in the following conditions:

   - Leakage of the dye, as is seen in choroidal neovascularisation (Figs. 3.13–3.15).This is one of the commonest indications for anti-VEGF intravitreal injections. Leakage can also be seen in cystoid macular oedema, which can occur following a branch or central retinal vein occlusion (Fig. 3.16). Similarly, diabetic macular oedema is characterised by diffuse hyperfluorescence (Fig. 3.17). Intravitreal anti-VEGF or steroid injections may be used to treat these conditions as well.
   - "Window defects" refers to areas where choroidal fluorescence becomes more visible owing to a defect in the RPE. This can be seen in areas of RPE atrophy secondary to dry age-related macular degeneration (Figs. 3.18 and 3.19).
   - "Pooling" refers to accumulation of fluorescein dye into an anatomical space that may have increased in size owing to a pathological process. A common example is a retinal pigment epithelial detachment (PED), the mechanism of which has been discussed in the OCT section. On an FFA this presents as an early well-defined filling of fluorescein under the detached RPE, which does not change in size and intensity in the late stage (Figs. 3.9–3.12).

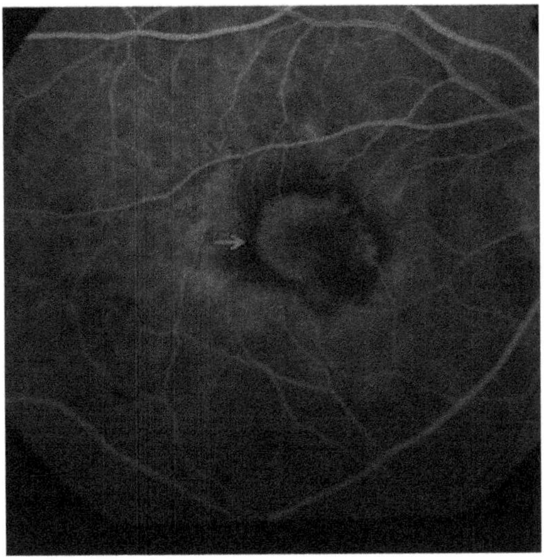

Fig. 3.13. An FFA showing early hyperfluorescence (within 30 sec) indicative of "classic" choroidal neovascularisation. The appearance is often described as having a "lacy" pattern.

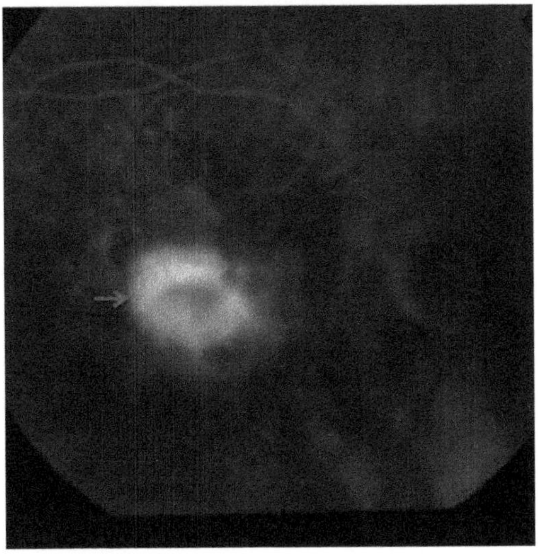

Fig. 3.14. An FFA of the same eye, showing increase in intensity and size of the hyperfluorescent area in the late phase (at 3 min). This confirms the presence of "classic" choroidal neovascularisation.

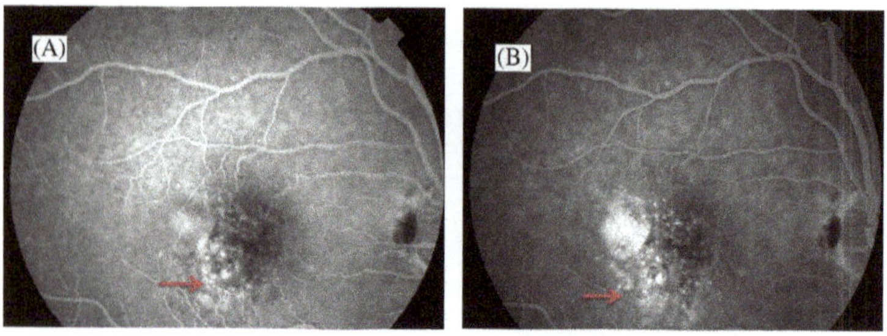

Fig. 3.15. An FFA showing late hyperfluorescence at approximately 40 sec, as indicated by the red arrow (image A). The area increases in intensity and size in the late phase at approximately 3 min (image B). The appearance is "stippled" and this is characteristic of "occult" choroidal neovascularisation.

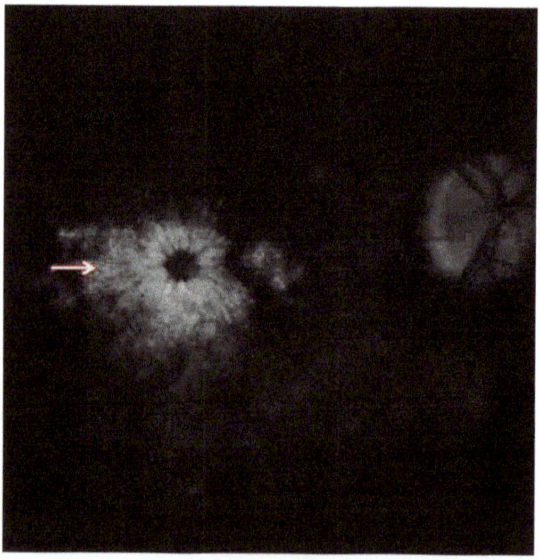

Fig. 3.16. An FFA showing late hyperfluorescence (at 6 min) in a "petalloid" pattern. This is characteristic of cystoid macular oedema.

Fig. 3.17. The FFA late phase (approximately 6 min), showing diffuse hyperfluorescence in a diabetic patient. This is indicative of diabetic macular oedema (area within red arrows).

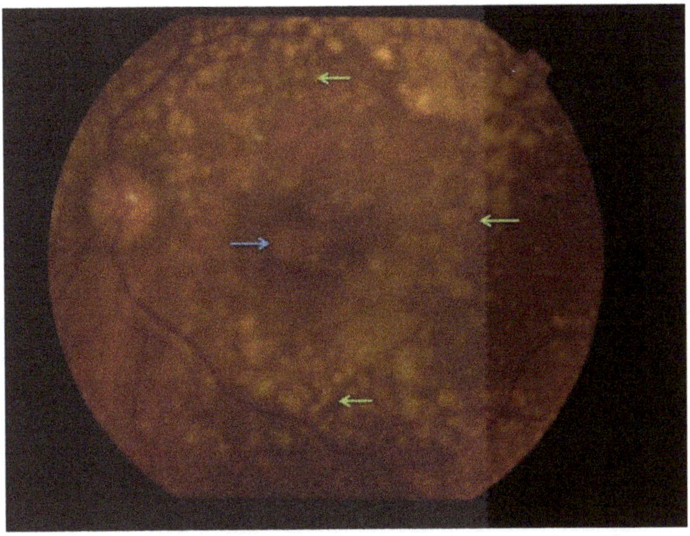

Fig. 3.18. A colour fundus photograph showing the central area of RPE atrophy (blue arrow) with numerous scattered drusen (green arrows).

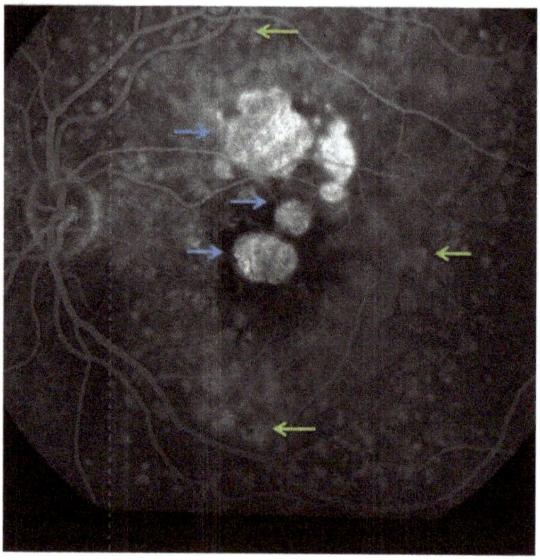

Fig. 3.19. The FFA late phase (3 min) of the same eye, demonstrating a window defect (blue arrows) alongside staining of drusen (green arrows).

- "Staining" refers to deposition of fluorescein dye within the involved tissue and occurs in both normal and pathological states. Normal structures such as the optic disc and sclera may stain. Pathological changes such as drusen and disciform scars can also show staining (Figs. 3.18 and 3.19).

Areas of hypofluorescence are seen in the following situations:

- Blockage or masking can be seen owing to bleeding within the retina. The major retinal vessels run within the nerve fibre layer, and the smaller capillaries in the inner nuclear layer. Thus, a retinal haemorrhage within the nerve fibre layer will block fluorescence from all the retinal blood vessels whilst one deeper in the retina will block only the capillary fluorescence (Figs. 3.20 and 3.21).
- Vascular filling defects are defined as areas of decreased blood supply which may be seen in conditions like diabetes and arterial occlusions.

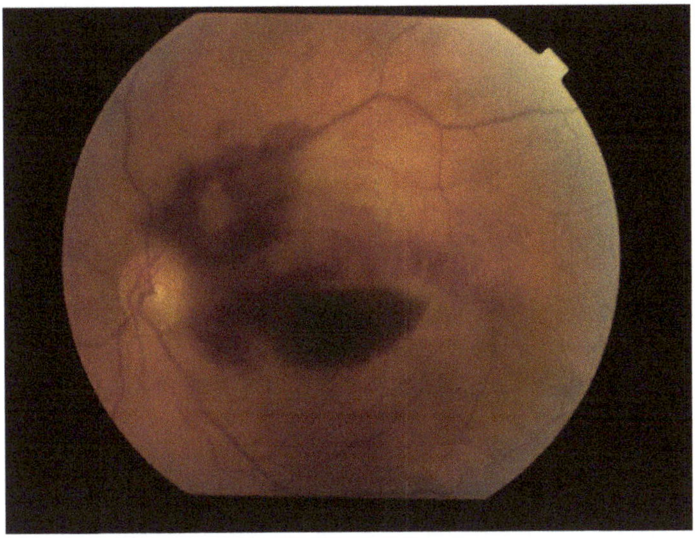

Fig. 3.20. A retinal haemorrhage.

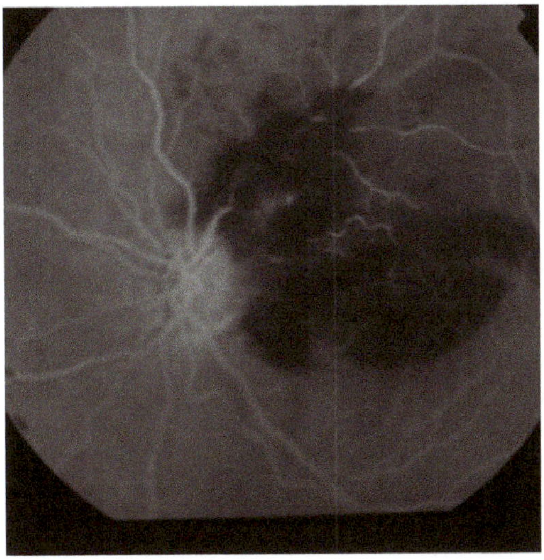

Fig. 3.21. The corresponding FFA, showing masking of fluorescence from both retinal and choroidal vasculature in the area of haemorrhage.

Points to remember

1. There is no evidence of increased incidence of anaphylaxis to fluorescein in patients with a history of anaphylaxis to other drugs or atopy.
2. There is no reported correlation between old age and incidence of adverse reactions (the oldest reported FFA is in a 98-year-old patient).
3. FFA is safe in patients on multiple drugs with no reported adverse reactions due to drug interactions.
4. Hepatic and renal failures are not contraindications to FFA. This is because in such circumstances the plasma half-life of a given dose of fluorescein is prolonged but the peak levels stay the same. Since fluorescein is given only once, there is no risk of cumulative drug toxicity.
5. There are no reports of damage to a pregnant woman or a foetus with fluorescein. However, pregnancy is a relative contraindication and FFA should be avoided unless absolutely necessary, particularly in the first trimester.
6. Fluorescein is excreted for up to four days in breast milk. Thus, breast feeding should be avoided for this duration. During this time women should use a breast pump and discard the milk.
7. There is no evidence of increased incidence of serious adverse events with uncontrolled diabetes or hypertension.

Further reading

We would recommend the following article, which we have referenced as well:

Mishra S, Al-Nuaimi D, Mclauchlan R, Mahmood S (Dec 2012/Jan 2013). Fluorescein angiography: safety issues and misconceptions *Eye News*.

OPTICAL COHERENCE TOMOGRAPHY ANGIOGRAPHY (OCTA)

This is a non-invasive approach that allows visualisation of retinal and choroidal blood vessels down to the capillary level. Although conventional OCT aids the clinician in detecting anatomic changes that impact vision, it cannot help contrast small blood vessels and static retinal tissue. Thus, it cannot be used to identify vascular changes such as pathologic new vessel growth in AMD or capillary drop-out (non-perfusion) in diabetic retinopathy. Traditionally these changes are detected by using either FFA or indocyanine green angiography (ICGA), but now OCTA has been developed as an extension of traditional OCT to allow a no-injection, dye-free method of looking at the ocular vasculature. In simple terms, it works by assessing the changes in the OCT signal caused by flowing blood cells and then presents this information to the clinician in a format that can be analysed.

Whilst the technology is still in its early stages and its exact place in clinical pathways is yet to be determined, it does offer the possibility of diagnosing most conditions, which previously required an FFA (Figs. 3.22 and 3.23). The big difference is that, with OCTA, the patient simply sits on an OCT machine and has some pictures taken (no injection of dye is required).

Further reading

You can find out more about this exciting new imaging modality by reading the following article, which we have referenced too:

Gao SS *et al.* (2016). Optical coherence tomography angiography. *Invest Ophthalmol Vis Sci.* **57**: OCT27–OCT36.

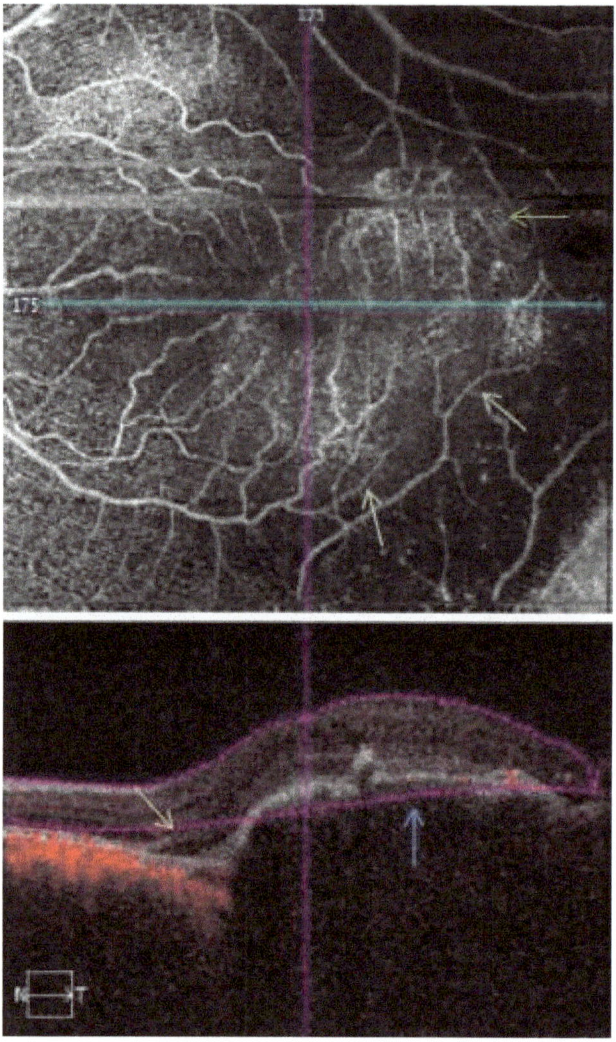

Fig. 3.22. OCTA showing an area of choroidal neovascularisation (green arrows in top image). The corresponding OCT shows a pigment epithelial detachment (blue arrow) and sub-retinal fluid (orange arrow). This patient has occult choroidal neovascularisation (confirmed on FFA).

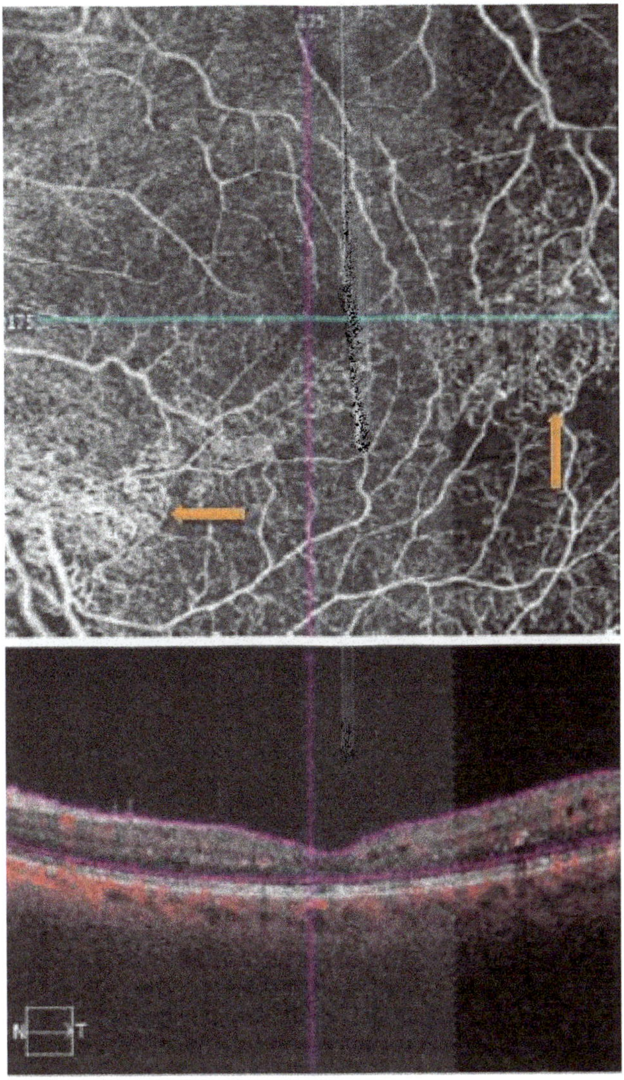

Fig. 3.23. OCTA showing collateral blood vessels in a patient with a branch retinal vein occlusion (orange arrows in top image). The corresponding OCT (bottom image) demonstrates absence of cystoid macular oedema.

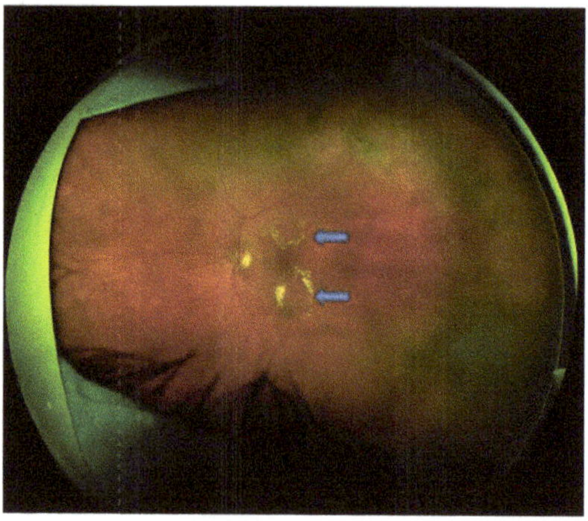

Fig. 3.24. A UWF colour fundus photograph of the left eye of a diabetic patient, showing areas of exudate within the macula (blue arrows). Note that the retinal periphery shows no abnormality.

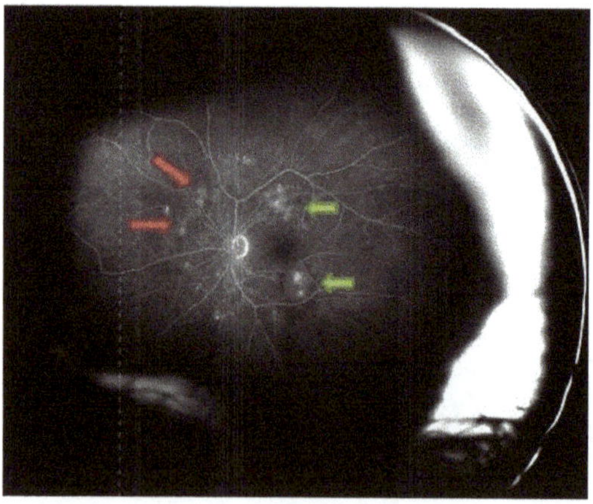

Fig. 3.25. UWF fundus fluorescein angiography of the same eye, showing macular oedema in the same locations (green arrows). Note that there are some other areas of oedema nasally as well (red arrows).

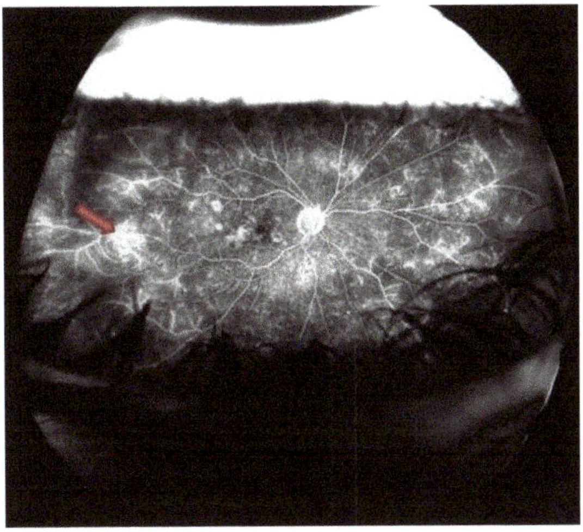

Fig. 3.26. UWF fundus fluorescein angiography of the right eye in a diabetic patient, showing peripheral neovascularisation (red arrow). This patient required laser treatment (pan-retinal photocoagulation) to halt further development of these abnormal blood vessels (which can cause vitreous haemorrhage and tractional retinal detachment).

ULTRA-WIDEFIELD IMAGING (UWF)

Conventional retinal imaging can only visualise approximately 30 degrees of the central retina. New ultra-widefield systems can now allow a fantastic 120-degree view of the retina, thus enabling better assessment of not only central but also peripheral retinal pathology (this view covers over 85% of the retinal surface). Current platforms are able to provide colour fundus photographs, fluorescein and indocyanine green angiograms, and auto-fluorescence images (Figs. 3.24 to 3.26).

4

INTRAVITREAL MEDICATIONS AND COMMON TREATMENT PATHWAYS

There are three common macular problems, which often require regular intravitreal therapy:

1. Wet age-related macular degeneration (AMD)–choroidal neovascular membrane (CNVM);
2. Diabetic macular oedema (DMO);
3. Retinal vein occlusion (RVO) with macular oedema.

For patients with wet AMD, the first-line treatment is typically a course of intravitreal anti-VEGF (antivascular endothelial growth factor) with aflibercept (Eylea), ranibizumab (Lucentis) or bevacizumab (Avastin). In some situations, such as when polypoidal choroidal vasculopathy is noted, photodynamic therapy (PDT) or thermal focal laser can also be indicated.

For patients with DMO, if the central retinal thickness is over 400 microns, then NICE (National Institute of Clinical Excellence) currently recommend considering a course of anti-VEGF injections. The alternative option is thermal laser (focal, grid or micropulse) or intravitreal steroid treatment. Intravitreal steroids for DMO that are currently available as sustained release depots are Ozurdex (lasting 4–6 months) and Illuvien (lasting 3 years). Intravitreal steroids cause cataract, so they are typically used only in patients who have had previous cataract surgery (are pseudophakic). They also carry a low risk of increasing the eye pressure (ocular hypertension; if untreated this can cause glaucoma). Unlike anti-VEGF, there are currently no concerns that intravitreal steroids may cause stroke.

For patients with RVO and macular oedema it is important to establish if the patient has a branch retinal vein occlusion (BRVO), a hemiretinal vein occlusion (HRVO) or a central retinal vein occlusion (CRVO). Patients with CRVO and macular oedema do not respond to macular laser and treatment options can include either an anti-VEGF course (often first-line) or an intravitreal steroid (usually second-line). Patients with BRVO can improve with macular laser, so this should remain as a treatment option for them — but often the results from laser are not as good as the results from the more invasive option of intravitreal anti-VEGF or intravitreal steroid. Patients with HRVO and macular oedema are less likely to respond to macular laser than patients with BRVO, but this could be tried if there was a contraindication to either anti-VEGF or intravitreal steroid.

WHAT ARE THE DIFFERENT ANTI-VEGF PATIENT PATHWAYS?

The problem with intravitreal pharmacotherapy is that the effect of the drugs will wear off after some time. It is important to explain to patients that their condition requires a "course" of treatment with ongoing injection treatments.

The different pathways available include a "loading phase" where injections are given reasonably often to try to stabilise or improve the patient's condition, and once they have reached a plateau (i.e. they are as well as they can get) treatment continues in a "maintenance phase" to keep them at that level of stability.

The aim is to give the patient as few injections as possible whilst ensuring that maximum visual function is achieved. The secondary aim is to minimise the number of patient visits so as to reduce the risk of patient fatigue (which results in reduced compliance and missed visits) and to maximise hospital eye service capacity.

The main different patient pathways available are:

1. Fixed Dosing

When anti-VEGF studies were introduced into research studies, patients were initially given the drug every month for 1–2 years. The outcomes were good and since then, in real-life scenarios outside of research trials, some units have adopted this fixed dosing pathway. Although the outcomes overall are good, the main problem with this approach is that some patients do not need this frequency of injections. Indeed, sometimes a patient may have only two loading injections and then not need a further injection for 3–4 months. If that same patient had been committed to a fixed dosing pathway, they would have had many more injections than they needed, which is not only an expensive use of resources but exposes the patient to the risk of the injection procedure (such as endophthalmitis) more often than is required. Some units still use fixed dosing pathways and try to find a balance by injecting eight-weekly rather than monthly; however, this carries the risk of under-treating those patients who do require the drug more often.

2. PRN

PRN ("*pro re nata*") means "as required" in Latin. It represents a shift from the fixed dosing schedule above to giving the injection only if the disease shows signs of activity. The benefit of PRN over fixed dosing is a likely reduction in the number of injections. The number of visits may be quite similar, since the patient still needs to attend for review for the possibility of having an injection. The problem with the PRN approach is that if time is spent waiting for disease activity to manifest, then some visual function may be compromised. For example, consider the patient who relapses at week 6 following their last injection. If they are coming monthly on the PRN pathway (and being injected only if signs of activity are present), then at their visit four weeks after their injection they will be "stable" and no injection will be given. Two weeks later, when they reach week 6, the disease activates and vision is lost, and the process to structural macular damage begins. However, the patient has to wait a further two weeks (or call as an emergency) until their next monthly visit. At this review, now eight weeks from their last injection, the PRN pathway allows an injection and both doctor and patient hope for recovery from the drop in vision and macular changes. Another problem with the PRN approach is the uncertainty that the patient has at each visit. For some patients, not knowing if they will or will not have an injection until the day of review causes significant anxiety, and also potential transport issues if they have to wait for treatment at a one-stop clinic.

3. Treat and Extend

The concept of the treat-and-extend pathway is to try to tailor the treatment to that individual patient so as to ensure that vision is maintained and the macula remains "dry" (or at the best plateau possible) with the minimum number of injections and visits. It is called "treat and extend" since at each visit the patient is treated and, if stable, an attempt is made to extend the gap between visits.

Patients typically receive loading injections as usual (for example, three monthly injections) and then for the next two or three visits initially start off on the PRN pathway (see above). Depending upon how the condition progresses during this period, it is usually possible to establish the time from the last injection at which the condition starts to reactivate. For example, if after the third loading injection, at the next monthly clinic review the macula is dry, on the PRN pathway, no injection will be given. If the patient then finds that three weeks later the vision drops (i.e. seven weeks from the last injection), then at their next review one option to consider is to treat the patient and then book them for a treat-and-extend appointment for seven weeks (i.e. the appointment time is booked to match the time of anticipated reactivation). At this seven weeks appointment they will be assessed (history, VA, fundoscopy, OCT), and if the condition is stable they will still be given an injection (hence a dry macula is still injected) and a plan to see the patient in 8–9 weeks made on the treat-and-extend pathway (i.e. at that visit in 8–9 weeks they will be injected and a review of the next timescale made). If at the seven weeks appointment the patient has reactivated and gives a history that the vision has dropped over the past week, then on the treat-and-extend pathway the patient will be injected but the next appointment for injection and review will be reduced from seven weeks to six.

Therefore, on the treat-and-extend pathway, the patient is injected (treated) at each visit and the main clinical decision to make is to either extend the duration between visits (if the patient is stable) or reduce the duration between visits (if the patient is unstable).

The benefits of the treat-and-extend pathway include the ability to keep the patient in the plateau phase without having to reduce visual function and lose macular anatomical integrity (which is required to allow treatment on the contrasting PRN pathway). It also reduces the number of visits for the patient and removes anxiety relating to the visit — since an injection is given each time. For some stable patients it becomes possible to extend the duration between injections or visits to 14 weeks. Once this target is reached it is possible to consider stopping treatment and observing for relapse.

4. Individualised Patient Treatment

As described above, the three main different pathways (fixed dosing, PRN, treat-and-extend) all have their benefits and problems. The favoured option should be the one that best matches the patient's individual circumstances. This will depend upon the frequency at which their disease reactivates and the ease with which they can attend the clinic.

From a capacity perspective, it is difficult for the hospital eye service to provide different pathways for different patients since it is easier logistically to adopt one pathway strategy for all patients. However, this results in over-treating some patients and under-treating others, and does not make an attempt to minimise patient visits depending upon their disease activity and their ability to come to the clinic.

The authors' preferred pathway is to have the flexibility to have the option to offer patients both the treat-and-extend and the PRN pathway depending upon their clinical situation. Although this creates logistical challenges for service provision, it does help to ensure the best care for our patients.

5

THE TECHNIQUE

The following is based on published guidance to reflect the latest clinical practice. There may be minor inter-departmental variations, although the general principles remain the same.

ONE-STOP AND TWO-STOP CLINICS

It is important to emphasise here that the technique described below is for a "one-stop" clinic where the clinician reviews the patient and the injection is delivered by a nurse practitioner straightaway. In this scenario the pre-injection checks outlined in Appendix C will already have been done by the clinician, and the nurse practitioner will simply have to fill in the section relating to the injecting process itself (please remember that the allergy, consent and correct eye marked should be checked again by the nurse practitioner). In contrast, a "two-stop" process is where the patient is seen by the clinician and a decision made to treat. The patient is then booked onto a separate injection list usually within a week or two for the nurse practitioner to inject. In this scenario, the pre-injection checks have to be repeated by the practitioner on the day and so familiarity with how to do them is important. In the second scenario, it is also important for the nurse practitioner to make sure that a clinician responsible for the list is accessible in case a complication occurs.

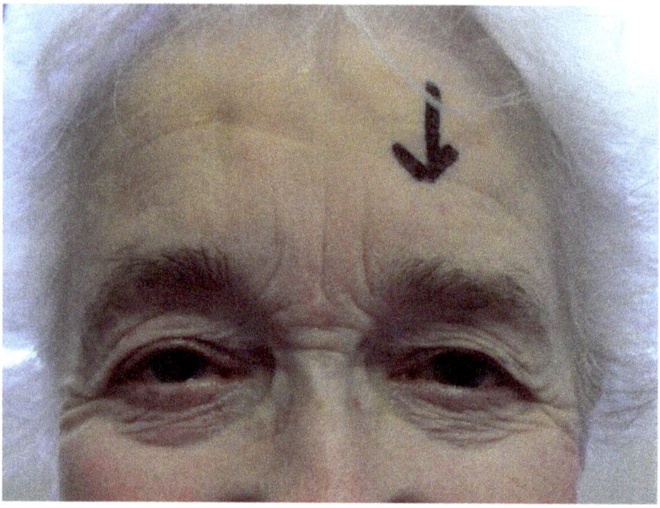

Fig. 5.1. Correct eye marked.

1. Confirm the identity of the patient with their notes (including name and date of birth). Do not proceed if the patient's notes are not available.
2. Confirm that the patient has signed a consent form and that they are able to confirm the eye that is to be treated. It is also essential to make sure that the eye to be injected has been marked by the clinician who saw the patient

NEAR-MISS SCENARIOS

These examples are worth remembering:

Two patients with the same name were in the waiting area. When the name was called, the wrong patient walked in, but because of the appropriate checks the error was picked up instantly and no harm done.

A clinician forgot to mark the eye to be injected in the clinic. This led to some confusion, and the nurse practitioner was about to inject the wrong eye. Thankfully, the patient pointed the error out and no harm was done.

(Fig. 5.1). Do not proceed if the consent form has not been completed or if there is confusion over which eye is to be treated.

3. Instil topical anaesthesia with proxymetacaine and tetracaine (Fig. 5.2), followed by 5% povidone–iodine, into the inferior fornix (Fig. 5.3). Instil proxymetacaine first, as this does not sting. It is very important to flood the eye (conjunctival sac) with iodine (do not simply clean the lids), since the commensal bacteria on the conjunctiva must be exposed to the iodine in order to kill them. Endophthalmitis following intravitreal injection is the most-feared complication, and the risk can be substantially

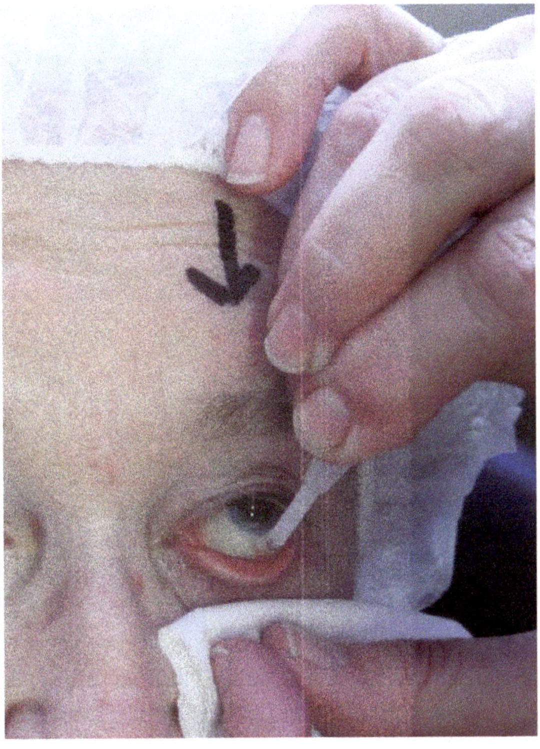

Fig. 5.2. Topical anaesthesia. Pulling the lower lid down exposes the inferior fornix, and the drops can be delivered here. When the patient blinks, the drops are distributed over the anterior surface of the eye.

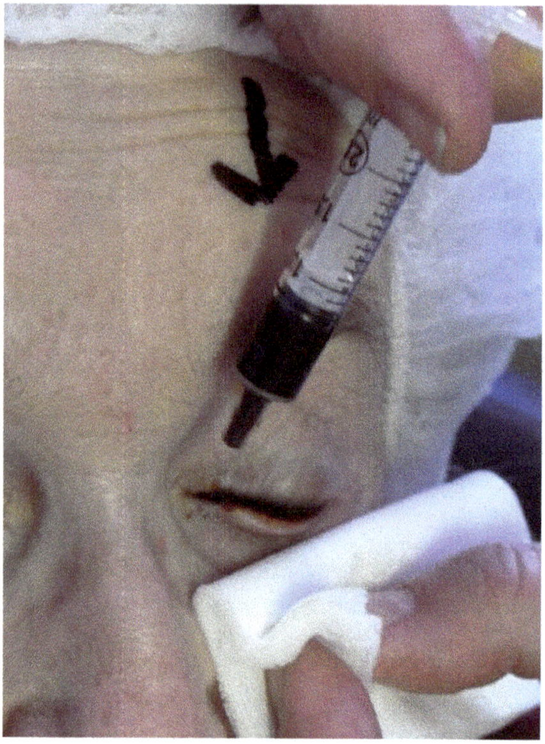

Fig. 5.3. 5% povidone–iodine to the inferior fornix.

CRITICAL INCIDENT

A patient developed a localised allergic reaction (swollen lid with itching) due to iodine use. This was documented, but iodine was inadvertently applied the next time as well. Thankfully, the allergy was localised and the patient recovered without any long-term sequelae. As an injection list can be very busy, this case highlights the need to double-check allergies (to iodine and to any antibiotics) with both the patient and the notes — "First, do no harm."

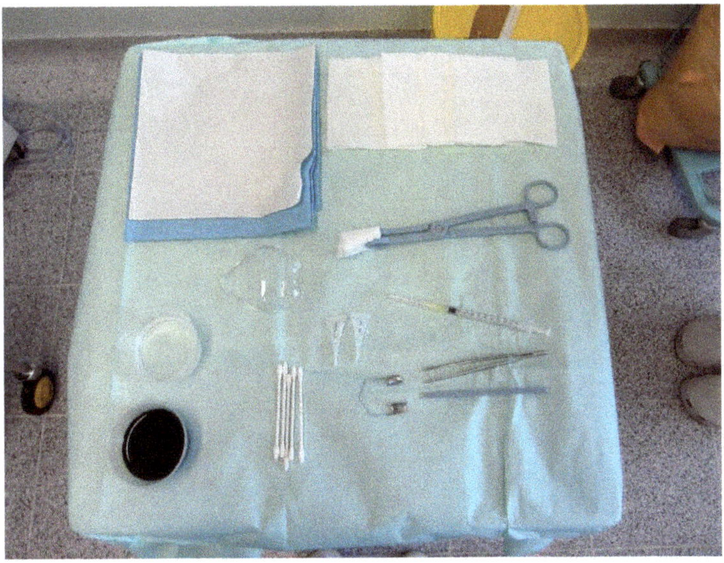

Fig. 5.4. Injection pack.

reduced with strict attention to the preparation of the injection site.

Note it is important to confirm whether or not the patient has any allergies prior to using iodine. If they are allergic to iodine, then an alternative aseptic solution must be used (usually aqueous chlorhexidine).

4. The practitioner is to wash their hands and use sterile gloves, and a hat and mask must be worn.
5. Set up the injecting kit (Fig. 5.4). Lucentis® comes preloaded in an injecting syringe, so place a 30-gauge precision glide needle and expel any excess without drawing back, such that 0.05 mL (which for Lucentis is equivalent to 0.5 mg) remains for injection. Avastin® and Eylea® need to be drawn up, so withdraw 0.2 mL through a large blunt filter needle into a 1 mL syringe, attach the aforementioned 30-gauge needle and expel any excess until 0.05 mL (which is equivalent to 1.25 mg for Avastin and 2.0 mg for Eylea)

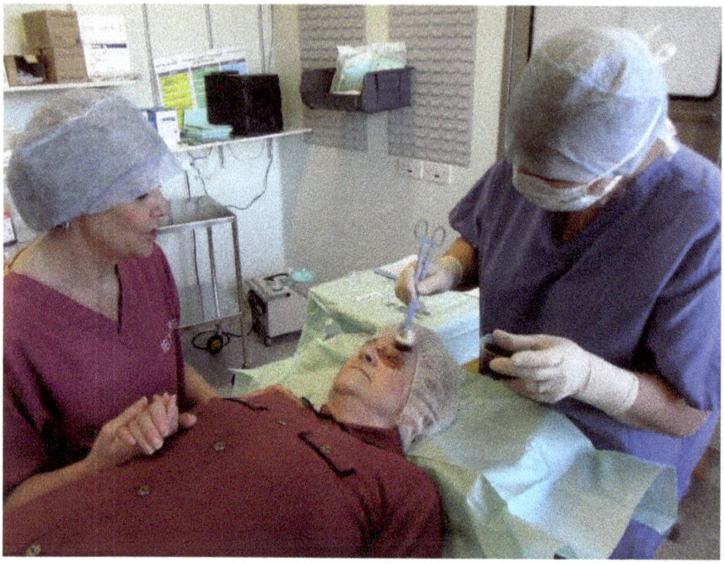

Fig. 5.5. 10% povidone-iodine prep prior to draping.

remains for injection. For all other intravitreal injections, the principle remains the same but it is important to make sure that the appropriate dose is being given.

6. Apply the full iodine preparation (10% povidone-iodine skin preparation) to the lids and surrounding skin prior to draping (Fig. 5.5). Remember that 5% povidone-iodine should already have been applied to the conjunctival sac and left for 3 min to ensure eradication of all conjunctival bacterial flora (as described in step 3). This is a vital step in order to reduce the risk of endophthalmitis. If this has not already been done, then ensure that it is completed before proceeding any further.
7. Apply a sterile drape and a sterile speculum (Figs. 5.6 and 5.7).
8. Ask the patient to look at the corner opposite where you plan to inject. For example, if planning to inject in the superotemporal quadrant, ask the patient to look down and in (inferonasally). In the quadrant where you plan to inject, measure the pars planar injection site 4 mm back from the limbus in phakic eyes (eyes that have their natural lens and

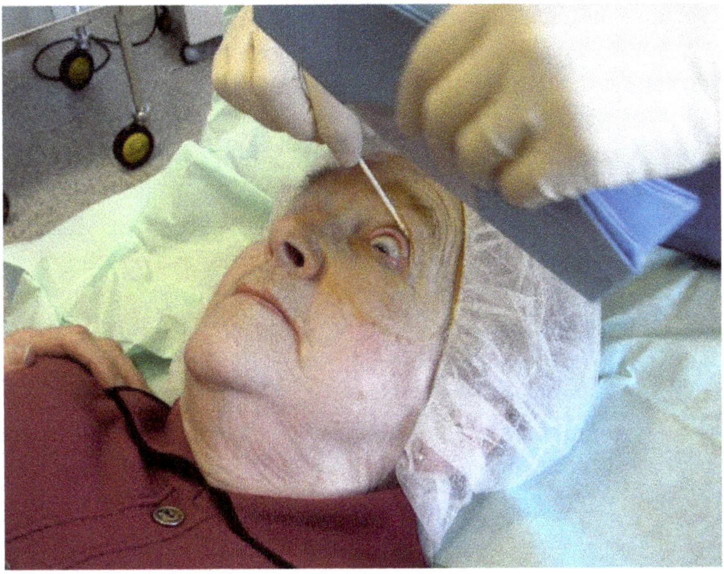

Fig. 5.6. The correct drape technique — ask the patient to look at their feet whilst exerting traction on the upper lid. This will allow the drape to engage the upper lid lash and avoid touch with the injecting needle.

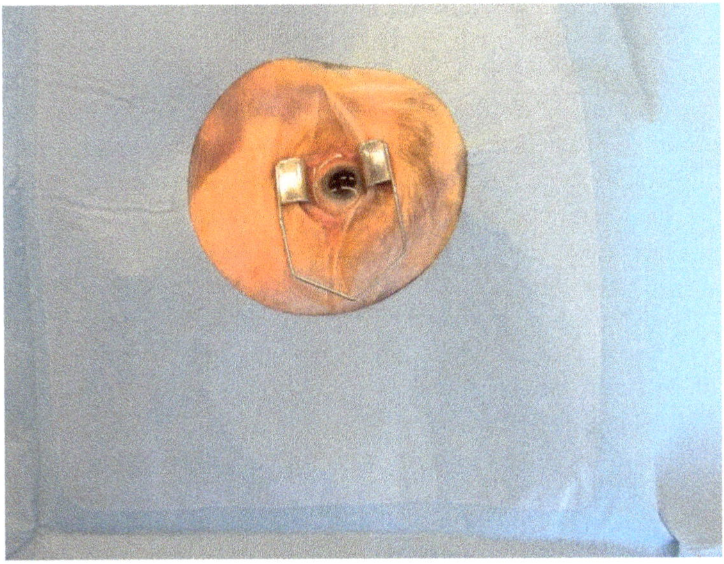

Fig. 5.7. Drape and sterile speculum correctly in place.

have not had cataract surgery) or 3.5 mm back from the limbus in aphakic/pseudophakic eyes (those that have no lens or have had cataract surgery and now have an artificial intraocular lens).

Angle the needle posteriorly and aim so that the needle is perpendicular (at a right angle) to the surface of the eye whilst also directed towards the central core of the vitreous. Using the correct entry point and correct angle will ensure that the needle passes safely through the pars plana and into the vitreous cavity without damaging the lens or the retina. If the needle is too close to the limbus or is angled too close to the lens, then it will touch the lens and cause a traumatic cataract. If the needle is too far away from the limbus, then it will pass through the retina and cause a retinal tear and retinal detachment. Also avoid contact with the lid margin (to reduce contamination of the needle with any possible bacteria). The bevel of the needle should be facing upwards. Sliding the conjunctiva circumferentially so that the scleral entry point does not coincide with the conjunctival entry point is advisable (so, after the injection has been completed, the conjunctiva will slide back and the hole in the conjunctiva will not lie directly over the hole in the sclera, theoretically reducing the risk of bacteria subsequently entering the eye).

9. Avoid three o'clock and nine o'clock injection sites, as the long ciliary nerves run in this position and can cause pain despite adequate topical anaesthesia. Also consider rotating quadrants when repeated injections are going to be needed, since thinning of the sclera can result from multiple injections. Some patients have pre-existing areas of scleral thinning which give a brownish hue owing to the visible underlying choroid. These should be avoided.
10. A sterile calliper should be used to measure the injection distance (Fig. 5.8).
11. Use a 30-gauge needle no longer than 15 mm to inject. Half to two-thirds of the needle is advanced into the eye (Fig. 5.9).
12. Inject the drug slowly over a few seconds. Then wait a few seconds more before removing the needle in a single

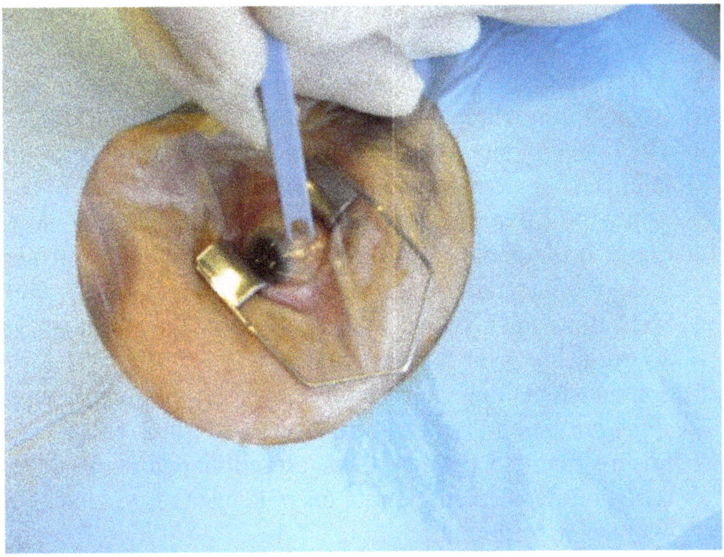

Fig. 5.8. Calliper to measure the distance from the limbus.

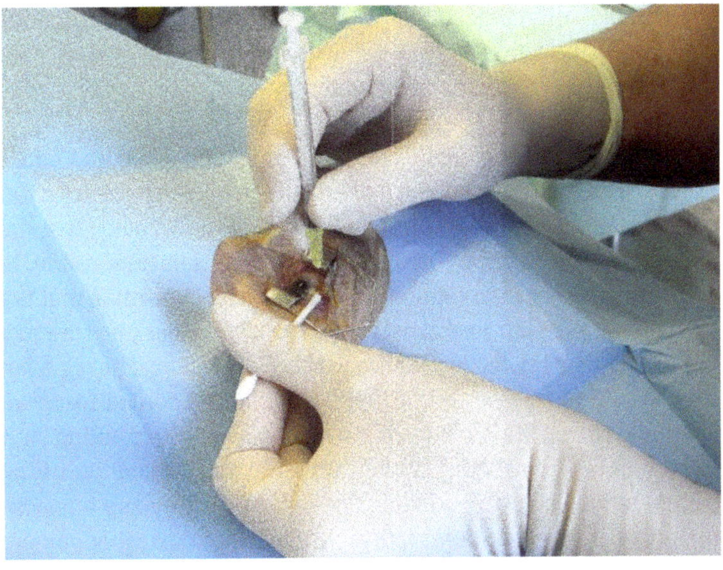

Fig. 5.9. Injection being delivered into the superotemporal quadrant.

controlled movement. This pause helps reduce the risk of drug reflux out of the injection site.

13. After removing the needle, apply a sterile cotton bud (soaked in povidone–iodine) to the entry site for 10 sec.
14. The injection site should be wiped radially away from the limbus, to remove any vitreous wick.
15. Apply topical antibiotics to the cornea and injection site.
16. Check if the patient can see and count their fingers at 1 m using the injected eye (by covering the other eye).
17. Some departments have a policy requiring the placement of an eye shield over the injected eye.
18. Some patients may be asked to have their intraocular pressures measured by the clinician post-injection.
19. Ensure that the patient has a prescription for antibiotics based on departmental preference. Remember to check for allergies to antibiotics.
20. Complete the intraocular procedure component of the patient pathway and ensure that the patient's name has been included in the intravitreal injection logbook. This is usually an A4-sized diary in which the patient's details, date of injection, name of medicine injected, eye injected and name of injector are documented.

Remember to document that the patient could see and count fingers with the injected eye post-treatment. In the event that a patient cannot see and count fingers with the treated eye, the patient must be taken immediately to the clinician responsible, to consider whether intervention is required. The concern is that the intravitreal injection may have raised the intraocular pressure to a high level, causing a central retinal artery occlusion. The clinician may decide to release fluid from the peripheral cornea using an insulin syringe, MVR blade or paracentesis blade, resulting in a rapid reduction in the intraocular pressure and restoration of the central retinal artery blood flow. Time is critical here and it is wise to always ensure that the responsible clinician knows that you are still injecting, so that they remain easily accessible. Also, it is sensible to check before every list where the required instruments are, so that valuable time is not lost searching for them.

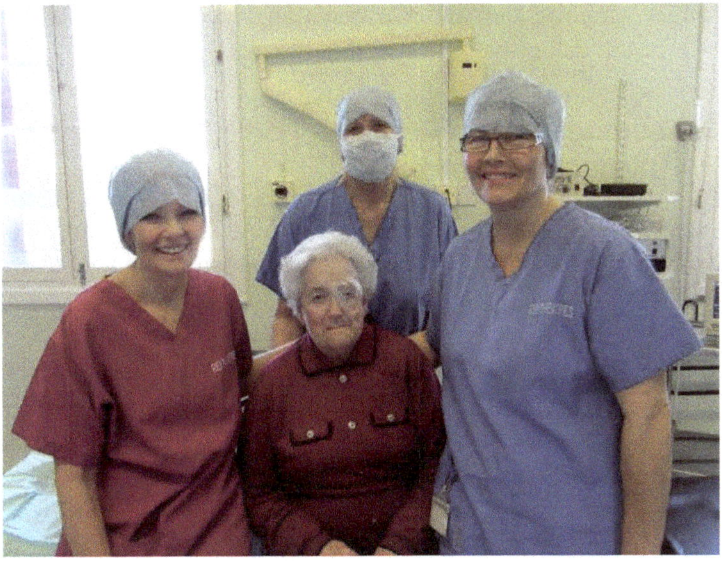

Fig. 5.10. A comfortable patient and a satisfied team at the end (Royal Eye Infirmary, Plymouth).

IMPORTANT POINTS TO REMEMBER

The following concepts will help in ensuring a competent intravitreal injection.

1. Effect of Positioning of the Eye

Ask the patient to look away from the quadrant you wish to inject and imagine where the centre of the eye is in relation to the injection point. If you enter perpendicular to the sclera here, the 15 mm needle cannot reach the opposite retina.

2. Positioning of the Needle in Relation to Ocular Structures

Any forward tilt of the needle will run the risk of lens damage. A backward or sideways tilt is safe as long as the needle does not go in completely. An oblique entry like this may theoretically reduce vitreous loss and the resulting longer track may also reduce the risk of bacteria entering the eye.

3. Thoroughness in Checking That It Is the Correct Patient and Correct Eye

Injection lists are typically busy, so there is a real danger of human error resulting in the incorrect patient or incorrect eye being injected.

4. Taking Care to Ensure That the Injection Site Is Prepared Meticulously with Povidone–Iodine

This is to reduce the risk of endophthalmitis. Remember of course that patients with ocular surface infections (such as conjunctivitis, microbial keratitis, uncontrolled blepharitis or nasolacrimal duct obstruction) should not have intravitreal injections since this will increase their risk of endophthalmitis. Therefore, if your patient has a red, irritable or watery eye prior to treatment, then you should not proceed until this is first addressed.

5. Other Pitfalls

Pathology in some quadrants may make the procedure more dangerous, e.g. tumours or previous retinal detachment surgery (which has involved buckles or bands placed around the eye).

6. Electronic Patient Record

Most hospitals now have an Electronic Patient Record (EPR) system in place. Remember that all the above-mentioned checks and tips for documentation remain the same, albeit in a different format on an EPR.

6

COMPLICATIONS

The reason why patients give their informed consent for an intravitreal injection is that, on balance, they perceive that the potential benefits of treatment outweigh the risks.

As with any surgical procedure, there is potential for complications at any stage and it is important for the practitioner to be aware of these.

WRONG PATIENT OR WRONG EYE INJECTED

There is a rapid turnover of patients receiving this treatment, so extra care is needed to ensure that the correct patient has the correct eye treated. All patients should have a mark over the eye to be injected. If both eyes are to be injected, then a mark over both is mandatory. Always confirm with the patient their name, date of birth and eye to be injected prior to proceeding.

IODINE USED IN A PATIENT WITH IODINE ALLERGY

Before instilling eye drops and cleaning with povidone–iodine, ask the patient if they have any allergies and cross-check this with the notes. Specifically, ask if they have had an iodine allergy in the past. Swelling of the lid, redness of the eye and excessive discomfort should raise concern about a localised allergy, and a doctor should be informed immediately. If the patient becomes systemically unwell (shortness of breath, collapse and rash), then follow the hospital's guideline for anaphylaxis.

PATIENT COLLAPSE

This may be due to the stress of the procedure exacerbating a patient's underlying medical condition (severe heart or lung disease). If a patient appears particularly unwell, then check with a doctor to see if the procedure is still necessary. Alternatively, collapse may be due to anaphylaxis to the iodine or intravitreal agent, in which case you should follow the hospital's guidance on anaphylaxis.

For any patient who collapses, call for help. Check for signs of life (pulse, breathing, movement). If there are no signs of life, immediately call the cardiac arrest team (dial 2222 — do not go through the switchboard, as this will take too long) and begin basic life support (chest compressions and ventilations) until those able to provide advanced life support arrive.

SUBCONJUNCTIVAL HAEMORRHAGE

This is a common but relatively minor complication, which occurs since the intravitreal injection needle must pass through the conjunctiva (Fig. 6.1). Patients on anti-platelet or anti-coagulation medication are at particular risk. If this occurs, explain to the patient that it should resolve in a week or so.

PROBLEMS ASSOCIATED WITH A DILATED PUPIL

In some susceptible individuals, dilating a pupil can cause the intra-ocular pressure to rise rapidly ("acute glaucoma"). This

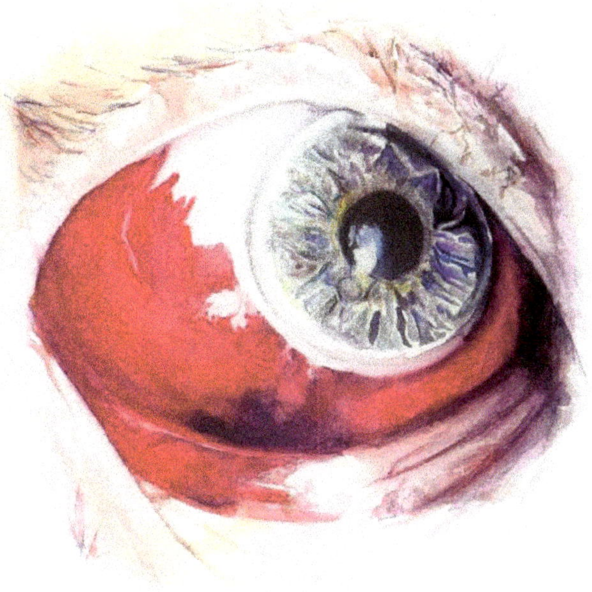

Fig. 6.1. Subconjunctival haemorrhage.

is more common in hypermetropes (long-sightedness) and the elderly, especially if there is a concurrent nuclear sclerotic cataract.

This risk is rare, and if there is concern it should be discussed with an ophthalmologist prior to dilating the pupil. There is no risk to patients with open angle glaucoma (the more common form of glaucoma) and the risk is present only for patients with narrow anterior chamber angles. However, eye clinic personnel need to be aware of this risk, and so if a patient reports pain or significantly blurred vision following the instillation of mydriatics, their eye pressure should be checked and a doctor informed.

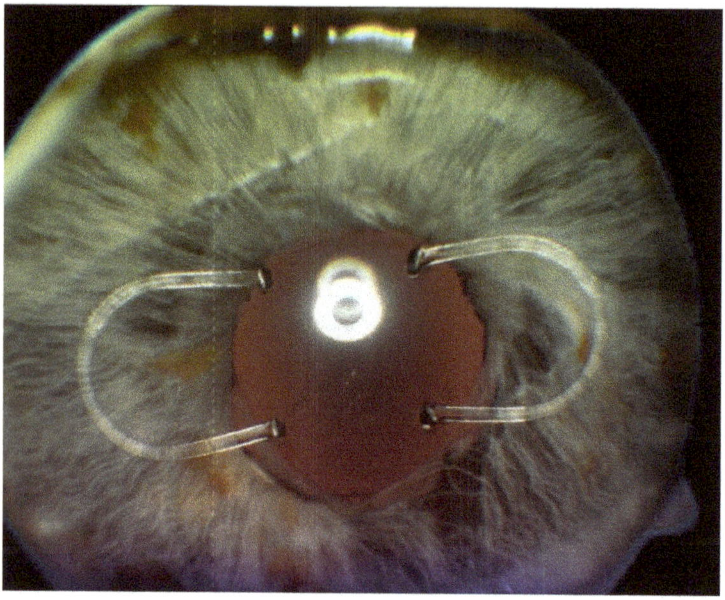

Fig. 6.2. A "lobster claw iris clip" lens. This was placed in patients with no capsular support to stabilise the lens (for example after intra-capsular cataract extraction). Dilation of the pupil may unhinge the clips, causing the lens to fall into the back of the eye. (*Photo courtesy of Mr Peter Simcock.*)

Some elderly patients may have had cataract surgery in the past with a "lobster claw iris clip" intraocular lens implant (Fig. 6.2). These patients should not be dilated. The patient will usually be aware of this and not let anybody dilate their eyes. Patients with artisan-style iris claw lenses can usually be safely dilated.

CORNEAL ABRASION

The cornea can be traumatised by the insertion of the speculum or a wayward needle. If it is damaged (Fig. 6.3), inform a doctor, who can assess further and consider additional treatment or altered follow-up.

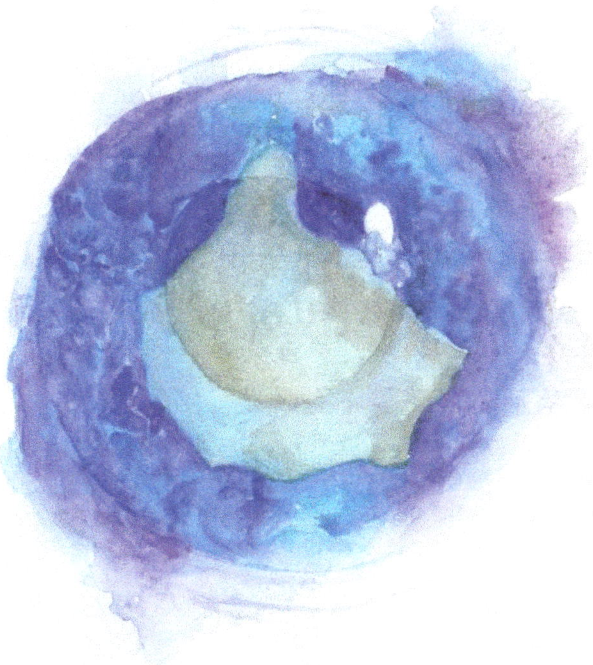

Fig. 6.3. Corneal abrasion showing fluorescein stain uptake (yellow-green area) when viewed using a blue filter on a slit lamp.

TOXIC EPITHELIOPATHY OF THE CORNEA

This occurs if excessive povidone-iodine or local anaesthetic affects the cornea, which is why we use lower-strength iodine. Always irrigate both the injection site and the cornea with a topical antibiotic after the procedure. Avoid priming syringes over the cornea.

CATARACT

If the intravitreal injection needle enters the eye too anteriorly or is angled too anteriorly, the lens can be damaged. This will result in a traumatic cataract and the patient may require cataract surgery. Traumatic cataracts can become manifest very quickly (same day) and are surgically complex to treat since the lens capsule will also be damaged. Managing traumatic cataracts is therefore more complicated and challenging than managing age-related cataracts. For this reason, it is important to be careful and always avoid lens touch with your needle.

POSTERIOR VITREOUS DETACHMENT AND RETINAL TEAR/DETACHMENT

An intravitreal injection can cause the posterior lining of the vitreous to detach from the retina. This in itself is usually harmless although the patient may notice more floaters. However, this process can also cause a retinal tear. Furthermore, if the intravitreal needle enters the eye too posteriorly or is angled too posteriorly, the retina can be torn. Failure to detect and treat a retinal

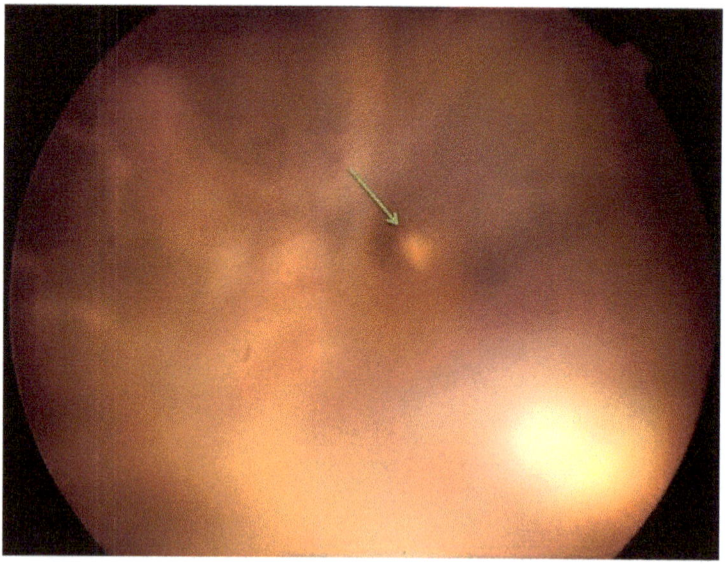

Fig. 6.4. Complete retinal detachment. Note that the retinal details are not clear and it looks elevated. The optic disc is barely visible (arrow). (*Photo courtesy of Dr Nalinda Samrakoon, Royal Eye Infirmary, Plymouth.*)

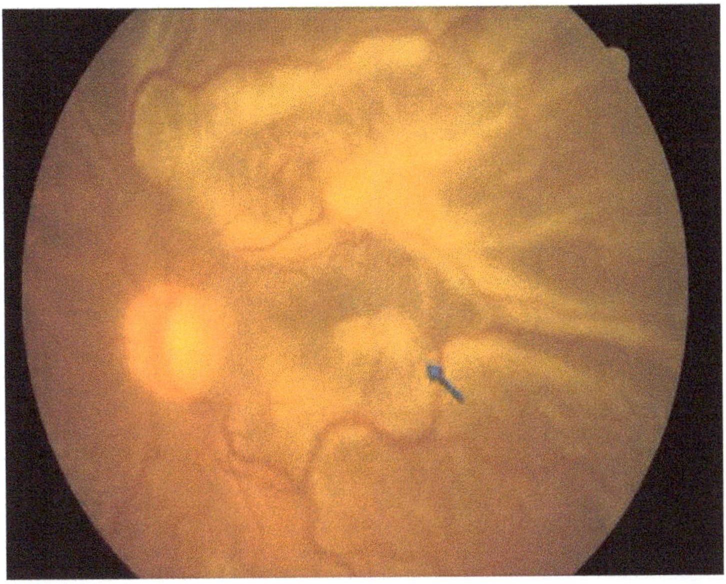

Fig. 6.5. A partial retinal detachment in the left eye (macula off). Note that the macula appears elevated with folds owing to underlying subretinal fluid (blue arrow). The optic disc and nasal retina appear intact. (*Photo courtesy of Mr Peter Simcock.*)

tear can result in the development of a retinal detachment (neurosensory retina peels off from the choroid), which causes permanent loss of vision if not detected and treated promptly.

RAISED INTRAOCULAR PRESSURE (IOP) / CENTRAL RETINAL ARTERY OCCLUSION / ISCHAEMIC OPTIC NEUROPATHY

If this occurs, it is usually transient and mild. However, if the patient has glaucoma or ocular hypertension, it may be necessary to check the IOP both before and after treatment that same day. Do ensure with a doctor that appropriate plans to check the IOP are made.

Rarely, the IOP can rise rapidly to very high levels. This can damage the retina (by causing a central retinal artery occlusion) or the optic nerve (ischaemic optic neuropathy).

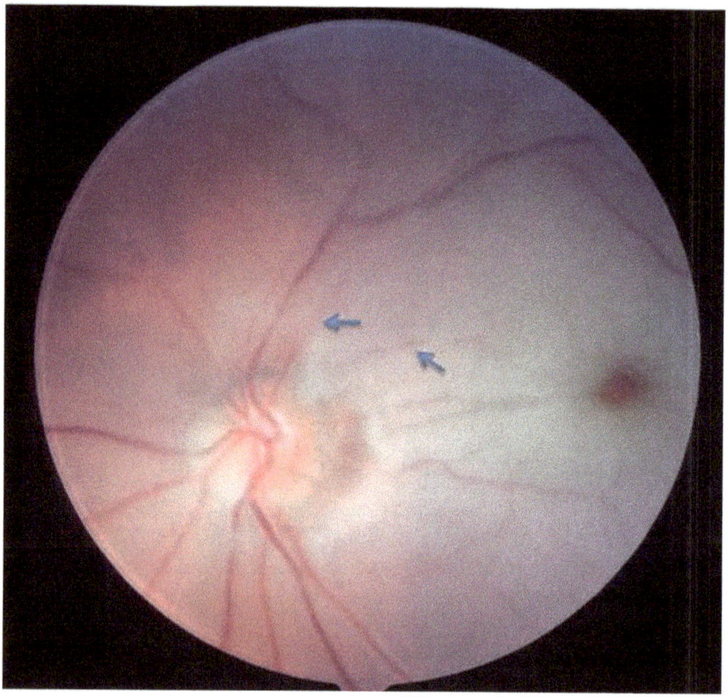

Fig. 6.6. A central retinal artery occlusion in the left eye. Note the generalised retinal pallor due to loss of blood supply. Note also the generalised thinning of the retinal arteries with segmented blood flow (blue arrows). (*Photo courtesy of Mr Peter Simcock.*)

For this reason, it is important to routinely check that the patient can see their fingers (counting fingers acuity) after the intravitreal injection. If the patient can do this, then such a high rise in the IOP is unlikely. If a patient cannot count their fingers after an intravitreal injection, then a doctor must be informed immediately and anterior chamber paracentesis considered.

AIR BUBBLES

When the drug is injected into the vitreous, there is a chance that air will also be injected inadvertently (usually trapped in the needle). This can cause more floaters than normal but usually resolves within a couple of days. If there is concern that a large amount of air may have entered the vitreous, then the intraocular pressure should be checked and discussed with a doctor.

VITREOUS WICKS

Sometimes, when the intravitreal needle is removed, vitreous may herniate through the scleral wound. This vitreous wick can act as a pathway for conjunctival bacteria to gain access to the vitreous cavity and cause endophthalmitis. Wait for a few seconds after the injection is complete to reduce reflux of the drug and remove the needle slowly. Put pressure on the injection site for 10 sec to reduce secondary vitreous loss. This complication can also be reduced by displacing the conjunctiva to one side before injecting, thus ensuring that the conjunctival entry point does not overlie the scleral entry point. Ten percent of injections are thought to leave some vitreous on the surface, which is why it is important to always use a sterile cotton tip and wipe away from the limbus over the injection site (once the needle is withdrawn).

ENDOPHTHALMITIS

This is perhaps the most devastating complication that can occur with intravitreal injections (Figs. 6.7 and 6.8). Endophthalmitis refers to a severe sight-threatening eye infection involving the vitreous cavity and anterior chamber. In addition to causing visual loss, severe cases unresponsive to treatment may require the eye to be eviscerated.

By ensuring adherence to a strict aseptic technique and appropriate storage of intravitreal agents, this risk is minimised to approximately 1 in 1,000 per injection. Patients should be aware of this risk and advised to contact the eye department immediately should they experience increasing eye pain, redness or deterioration in vision.

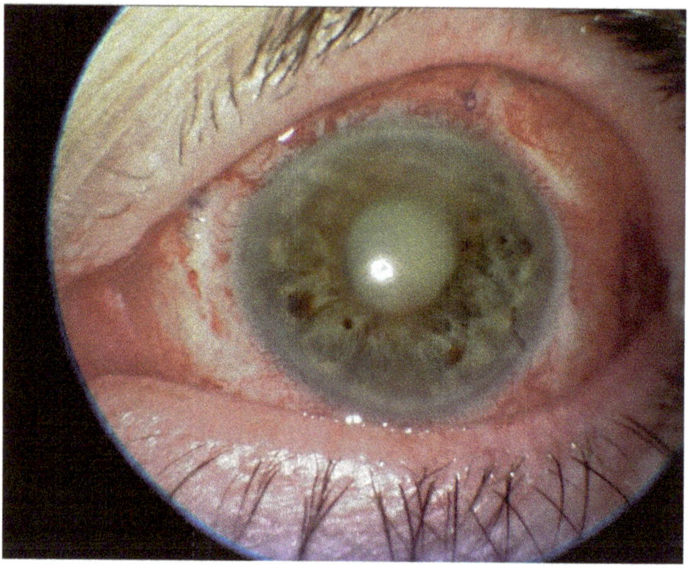

Fig. 6.7. Endophthalmitis. Note that the eye is inflamed, with an absent red reflex. Hypopyon (pus in the anterior chamber) is commonly seen but is absent in this eye.

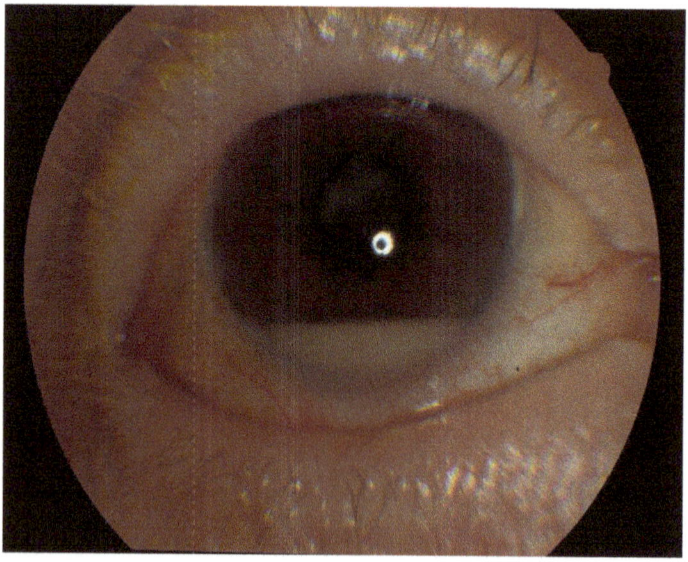

Fig. 6.8. An eye with endophthalmitis. Note the presence of pus in the anterior chamber (hypopyon). (*Photo courtesy of Mr Peter Simcock.*)

IMPORTANT STUDY

Post-intravitreal Anti-VEGF Endophthalmitis in the United Kingdom: Incidence, Features, Risk Factors and Outcomes

This was a prospective observational case control study performed by the British Ophthalmic Surveillance Unit (BOSU). Forty-seven cases of post-intravitreal anti-VEGF endophthalmitis (PIAE) were identified between January 2009 and March 2010 throughout the UK. Thus, the estimated incidence of PIAE was found to be 0.025%. The mean age of presentation was 78 years. The mean number of injections before PIAE was 5. The mean days to presentation was 5 (range 1–39). Positive microbiology cultures were obtained in 59.6% of cases, giving a culture positive incidence of 0.015%. The majority of causative organisms were gram-positive (92.8%). The most common presenting symptom was reduction in vision (96%), followed by pain/photophobia and redness. The most common signs were vitritis, hyperaemia and hypopyon. The majority of patients (63.6%) had worse vision after six months' follow-up when compared with acuity pre-PIAE.

Significant risk factors were:

1. Failure to administer topical antibiotic drops immediately after injection;
2. Blepharitis;
3. Subconjunctival anaesthesia;
4. Patient squeezing during injection;
5. Failure to administer topical antibiotics before anti-VEGF injection.

Recommendations made were:

1. Adequate treatment of blepharitis and eyelid check before injection;
2. Avoidance of subconjunctival anaesthesia if possible;

(*Continued*)

(Continued)

3. Administration of topical antibiotics immediately after injection;
4. To consider administering topical antibiotics before injection. This step was left to the discretion of the clinician.

The citation for the full paper is:

Iyall DAM *et al.* (2012). Post-intravitreal anti-VEGF endophthalmitis in the United Kingdom: incidence, features, risk factors and outcomes. *Eye* **26**: 1517–1526.

IMPORTANT: Do remember that most practitioners are very cautious as they start doing intravitreal injections. However, as experience is gained there is a risk of going into autopilot mode especially on high-volume lists, which may result in not every step being given appropriate attention, thus leading to complications. It is important to remember that each eye being injected is precious and only by giving every step of every injection due attention can complications be minimised.

Further reading

The following paper presents a good review of ocular and systemic complications associated with intravitreal anti-VEGF agents:

Falavarjani KG, Nguyen QD (2013). Adverse events and complications associated with intravitreal injection of anti-VEGF agents: a review of literature. *Eye* **27**: 787–794.

7

INJECTION DEVICES

Recently many innovative devices have become available on the market for precise and efficient delivery of intravitreal injections. To varying degrees, they obviate the need for a drape, speculum and calliper, thus making the injection process not only more comfortable for the patient but also safer in the hands of the practitioner.

MALOSA INTRAVITREAL INJECTION GUIDE (MALOSA MEDICAL/BEAVER-VISITEC INTERNATIONAL)

This guide is available as a single-use CE-marked and FDA-approved product worldwide, both on its own and as part of an injection pack. It consists of a triangular base plate which is curved to follow the contour of the eye and has three studs at the corners for stabilisation of the eye. Its apex has an arrow to indicate placement at the limbus. The base plate is connected to a cylindrical chamber, which in turn is connected to a handle and a lash guard. The lash guard is able to effectively splay the lashes away from the site of the injection and the injection needle (thus obviating the need for a speculum/drape whilst also reducing the risk of infection), and the cylindrical chamber allows 7 mm of a 13 mm/30-gauge needle to enter the eye (thus eliminating the risk of over-insertion). Once the base plate is firmly placed on the surface of the eye, the chamber will only allow the injection to be delivered 4 mm from the limbus, and perpendicular to the sclera, thereby ensuring precise delivery through the pars plana and avoiding lenticular/retinal damage. Concerns have been raised about the risk of particulate entry into the eye from plastic linings of needle chambers of injection devices. To negate this, a metal swage tube has been incorporated into the chamber as well. In addition, it has been developed by National Health Service innovation panels in Plymouth and Torbay, and thus for each unit used a proportion of the revenue generated comes back to the NHS.

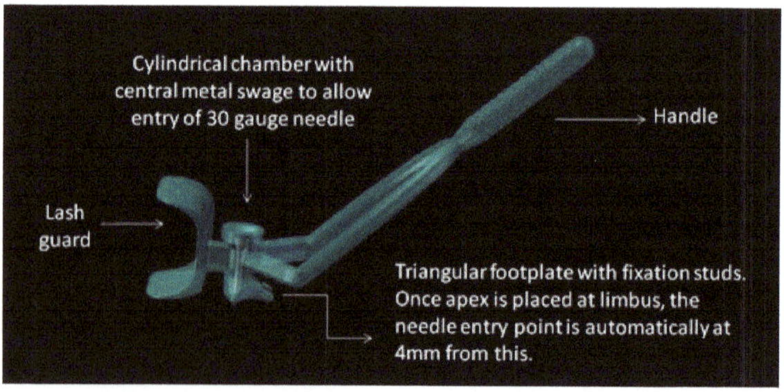

Fig. 7.1. The MALOSA Intravitreal Injection Guide.

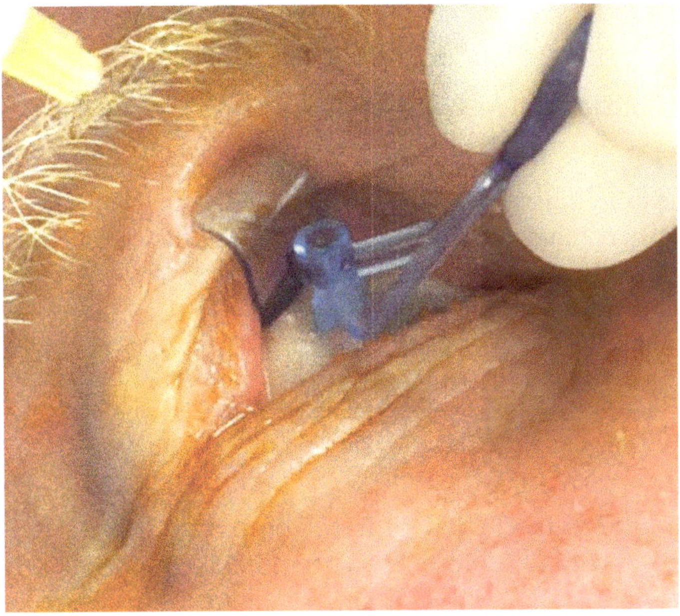

Fig. 7.2. Delivery of injection using the guide.

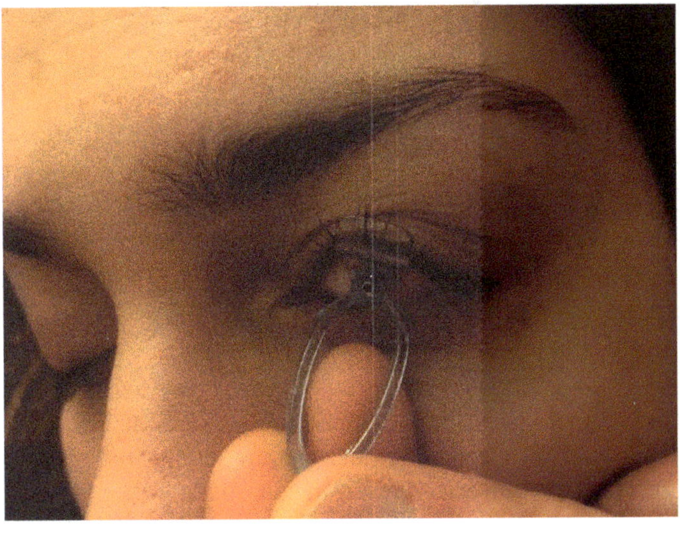

Fig. 7.3. Placement of guide on the ocular surface, showing the lashes neatly splayed out of the way.

CLINICAL EXPERIENCE

Retrospective Audit of 40 Cases

A retrospective audit of 40 cases performed at the Royal Eye Infirmary, Plymouth (UK) showed no complications (endophthalmitis/lens touch/retinal detachment/subconjunctival haemorrhage/corneal abrasion). Very positive patient feedback was received, in particular with regard to the elimination of drape and speculum. Our nurse practitioner found the guide very easy to use and commented that in difficult cases it was able to stabilise the eye very effectively, thus allowing delivery of a safe injection.

Randomised Control Trial Comparing Injection Using the Guide to the Standard Technique

Twenty-five patients at King Edward Medical University (Lahore, Pakistan) were randomised to injection using the guide, whilst 25 received it via the standard technique. Pain scores were recorded for both groups alongside complication rates. No complications were noted in either group. The pain score was found to be better in the guide group.

The results of both studies have been submitted for peer review and publication.

INVITREA (FCI OPHTHALMICS), SP.EYE (SD HEALTHCARE) AND RAVI GUIDE (KATALYST SURGICAL)

These devices also allow precise delivery of an intravitreal injection, albeit via different designs. In addition, SP.eye has a built-in safety feature to prevent needlestick injuries.

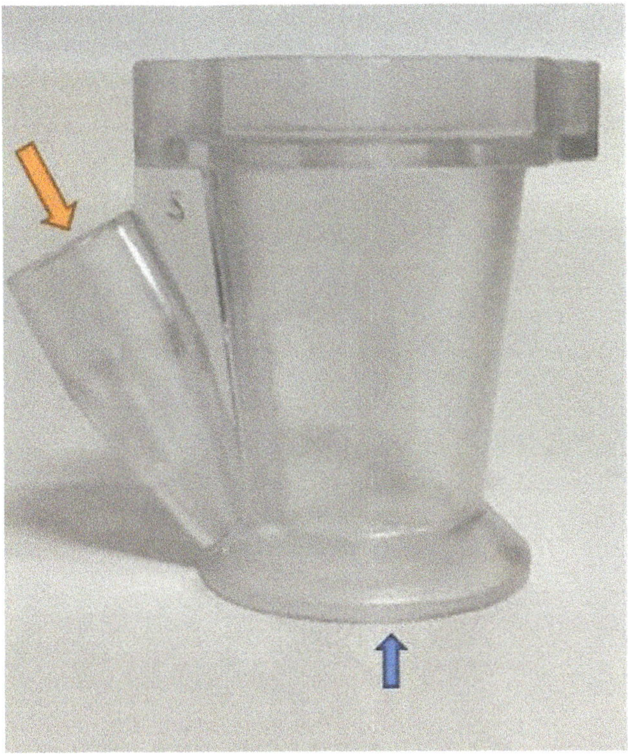

Fig. 7.4. InVitrea: Placement of the circumferential footplate on the limbus (blue arrow) allows delivery of the injection at the desired place via a side port (orange arrow).

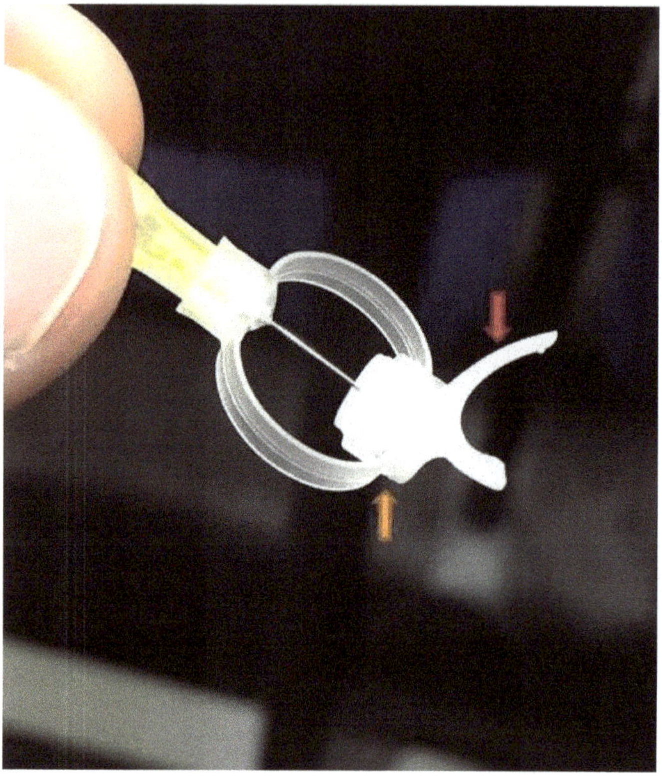

Fig. 7.5. SP.eye: the footplate (red arrow) is placed on the limbus. The chamber (orange arrow) includes a sharps safety mechanism.

8

PROTOTYPE TRAINING STRUCTURE

Proceeding with a specialised role can often be a daunting decision for nurses to make. However, once the decision has been made there may be further challenges ahead. In areas where nurses have only recently started to take on extended roles, training structures can be lacking. Intravitreal injection training at present has no defined curriculum by either the Royal College of Nursing or the Royal College of Ophthalmologists. It is thus left to the individual department to try to forge a training structure, which can be time-consuming. Here we outline a scheme we have used in our region over the last few years. The reader can feel free to adopt it in its entirety or modify it to suit their departmental needs. In our experience, both trainers and trainees have found it relevant and easy to undertake.

1. REQUIREMENTS FOR STAFF PERFORMING INTRAVITREAL INJECTIONS

1. Must be a registered ophthalmic nurse, optometrist or orthoptist.
2. Have done the ENB 346 course (Ophthalmic Nursing) or have equivalent orthoptic or optometric experience with a minimum of one year's consolidation.

3. Have a reasonable level of stereopsis.
4. Be experienced in other procedures that ensure a degree of manual dexterity (e.g. sub-Tenon's injections, botulinum toxin injections, incision and curettage of chalazia, electrolysis). Staff will also have to perform supervised "mock" intravitreal injections on pig eyes or plastic eyes.
5. Receive two tutorials from ophthalmic medical staff.
6. Review the basic knowledge in this handbook. All practitioners will be required to demonstrate background knowledge by obtaining at least 80% marks in an MCQ examination.
7. Complete a training programme with a consultant ophthalmologist or an experienced practitioner and obtain a certificate of accreditation.
8. Be observed performing 10 intravitreal injections by a second consultant ophthalmologist.

2. REASSESSMENT

Staff will require reassessment every year by a consultant ophthalmologist (three observed injections), at which point they will also have to produce evidence of ongoing learning, self-assessment and a logbook. If there is a lapse of clinical practice for 12 weeks or more, then reassessment by a consultant will also be required.

3. CLINICAL GOVERNANCE

The practitioner will keep a diary of all injections undertaken whilst under supervision. For the first 50 cases after accreditation, the consultant responsible will assess the patient one month later to check for complications. Outcomes will be reported in the diary.

During this period a protocol for pain assessment will be used to feed back patient satisfaction. Results will then be compared to a previous baseline audit of consultant practice.

A log of all injections will be kept as evidence for annual reassessments.

4. TRAINING PROGRAMME

The practitioner will be expected to read this handbook.

This basic knowledge will be reinforced with two one-hour tutorials describing the intravitreal injection technique by a consultant ophthalmologist.

There will be a multiple-choice questionnaire (20 key questions) in which the practitioner will have to score 80% correct (no negative marking).

The practitioner will then obtain the following practical experience:

1. The practitioner will observe 20 injections undertaken by a consultant ophthalmologist or an experienced senior practitioner.
2. The practitioner will then perform 50 intravitreal injections supervised by a consultant ophthalmologist or an experienced senior practitioner.
3. If that is satisfactory, the practitioner will perform unsupervised the next 20 cases.
4. There will be a final session once the practical sessions are completed to establish an audit process and patient satisfaction survey.
5. Once the practitioner has satisfactorily completed this training programme, they will have to inject 10 patients observed by a second independent clinician, in order to be finally accredited.

5. ACCREDITATION

The following competencies should be assessed at the end of the training period by a second independent clinician for accreditation:

1. Preparation and maintenance of the intravitreal injection room;
2. Understanding of the consenting process;

3. Understanding of the role of a supporting health care assistant;
4. Preparation of the patient and monitoring requirements.
5. Intravitreal injection (10 injections observed);
6. Post-injection assessment of the patients;
7. Understanding of complications and ability to identify when not to give an injection;
8. Management of complications and understanding when and how to call for help;
9. Post-injection patient instructions;
10. Procedure for responding to a patient collapse.

6. GUIDELINES FOR ASSESSORS

When undertaking instruction and assessment and before signing the certificate of competence, the assessors should satisfy themselves that the practitioners understand:

1. The anatomy of the eye and the orbit;
2. The issues of informed consent;
3. The preparation required;
4. Complications and how they are managed alongside the aftercare of a patient;
5. The management of a collapsed patient;
6. The appropriate documentation;
7. Audit and patient satisfaction survey procedures.

OUR EXPERIENCE

A Safety Audit of the first 10,000 Intravitreal Ranibizumab Injections Performed by Ophthalmic Nurse Practitioners

A prospective safety audit in our region found that carefully selected and well-trained nurse practitioners are

(*Continued*)

(*Continued*)

capable of delivering a safe and effective intravitreal injection treatment service. Two trained nurse practitioners administered 10,006 injections in the first 5.5 years of the service (1 May 2008 to 8 October 2013). This represented 84.1% of the total injections performed within the unit during the period. Four patients developed presumed infectious endophthalmitis (one was culture-positive and three were culture-negative). The incidence of post-injection endophthalmitis was therefore 0.04%, which compares favourably with the rate established by the British Ophthalmic Surveillance Unit. There was no evidence of lens touch, retinal detachment or systemic thromboembolic events. This work demonstrates how such a service can be established and provides safety data that other units can use as a benchmark when evaluating their own practice.

The citation for the full paper is:

Simcock P, Kingett B, Mann N, *et al.* (2014). A safety audit of the first 10,000 intravitreal ranibizumab injections performed by nurse practitioners. *Eye* **28**(10): 1161–1164.

IMPORTANT: Do ensure that both your trust and the Royal College of Nursing are happy with the medico-legal aspect of injection. Needless to say, this is important on the rare occasion where a complication results in a legal challenge. Your directorate manager can help clarify whether trust indemnity covers you for intravitreal injections and you can contact the Royal College of Nursing yourself for clarification.

9

SETTING UP A WETLAB

Organising a wetlab session can be invaluable for training to do intravitreal injections. This can easily be done by following the steps below:

1. Supervised “mock” intravitreal injections on pigs’ eyes are performed as per the technique described earlier.
2. Split pig heads (split down the middle, as shown in Figs. 9.1 and 9.2) can be easily acquired from your local butcher. We have used them very successfully in local courses for ophthalmologists and to train our nurse practitioners as well.
3. The pigs’ heads should be kept in a tray (as shown) to avoid spillage of fluids used.
4. The complete procedure can be easily practised, starting from draping all the way through to giving the injection.
5. Special care should be taken to dispose of the anatomical waste (i.e. pigs’ heads). Most hospitals require the use of yellow bin bags that have to be placed in special clinical waste collection areas. Do consult your hospital’s clinical waste disposal team for specific instructions.

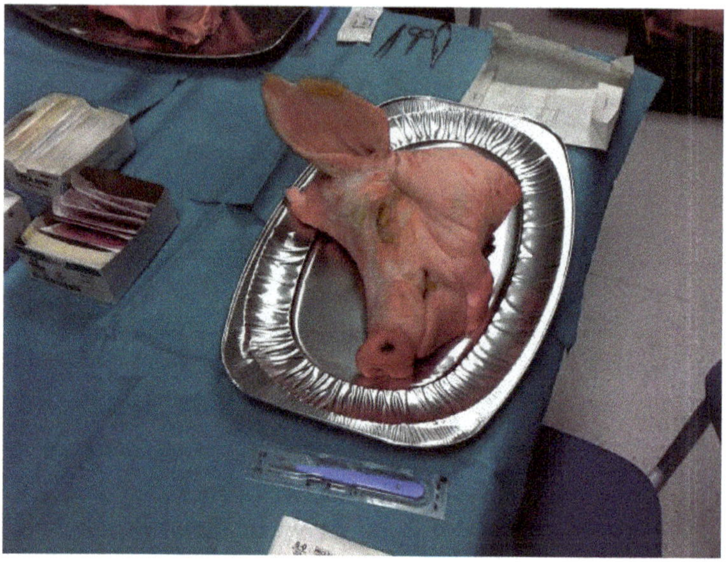

Fig. 9.1. A split pig head.

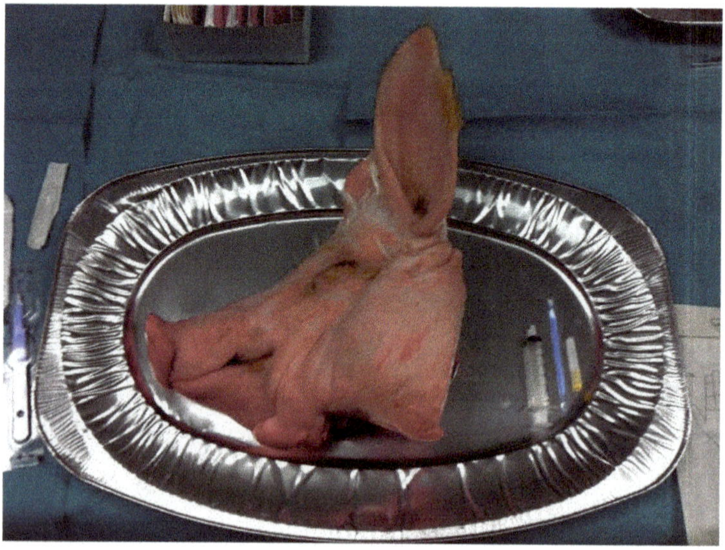

Fig. 9.2. A split pig head with injecting equipment.

10

ORGANISING A DEDICATED CLEAN ROOM

Intravitreal injections may be carried out in a theatre or in a dedicated clean room for outpatients. The volume of injections required on a daily basis in most eye units has led to the vast majority being done in outpatients. Whilst organising a clean room one must keep in mind the following precautions:

1. The room should deal only with non-infected cases and be free from interruptions. Check with your local infection control team regarding the exact specifications of a clean room in your hospital.
2. The room must have good illumination and washable floors (as confirmed by local health and safety regulations).
3. The ceiling should be non-particulate in nature, so that no dust or debris can fall onto the operating field.
4. Resuscitation facilities should be available nearby. The room should also have a reclining chair or a bed with an adjustable incline, so as to be able to change the patient's position in case an emergency occurs.

Further information can be found in the following resources:

1. *The Royal College of Ophthalmologists: Guidelines for Intravitreal Injections Procedure 2009.*
2. *Department of Health: Health Building Note 00–09. Infection Control in the Built Environment.* (Published March 2013.)

FURTHER READING

We recommend the following excellent textbooks:

1. Snell RS, Lemp MA (1997). *Clinical Anatomy of the Eye*, 2nd ed. Wiley-Blackwell.
2. Kanski JJ (2015). *Kanski's Clinical Ophthalmology: A Systematic Approach*, 8th ed. Saunders.

APPENDIX A: INTRAVITREAL INJECTION CHECKLIST

Patient's surname: First name: Hospital number: DOB: Affix patient label here if available

PRE-INJECTION ASSESSMENT

- **Allergies (including latex):**
- **Written consent:** Yes/No
- **Recent stroke/TIA:** Yes/No
- **Recent cardiac episode:** Yes/No
- **Current vision:** Rt: Lt:

- **Blepharitis:**
  Present: Treated with:
  Not present:
- **Regurgitation test (check for lacrimal sac collection):**
  Present: Treated with:
  Not present:
- **Correct eye marked:** Yes/No

RECORD OF PROCEDURE

Date:
Right/Left intravitreal (write name of drug):
Performed by: Injection no.:
Povidone–iodine/chlorhexidine prep:
Dose of injected drug:
Site of injection:
Can patient count fingers at end:
Complications:
Follow-up arrangements:

NOTES TO ASSIST PRE-INJECTION ASSESSMENT

Blepharitis. This is a chronic inflammatory condition of the eyelids. It is most commonly caused by a dysfunction of the oily glands in the lids (meibomian glands). This is called seborrheic blepharitis. It can also be caused by a mild bacterial infection (staphylococcal blepharitis), and sometimes the two forms coexist. Commonly seen signs are:

- Flaking, scaling and crusting around the eyelashes, like dandruff (Fig. A.1);
- Red eyelids, especially around the eyelashes;
- Soreness and irritation;
- In severe cases, small ulcers which can bleed can develop alongside the eyelashes.

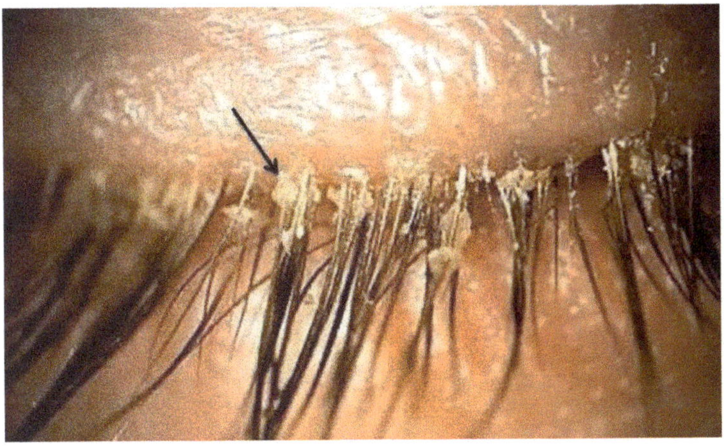

Fig. A.1. Blepharitis with crusting around the eyelashes (arrow).

An eye with blepharitis has a higher chance of developing endophthalmitis after an intravitreal injection, so it is important to recognise and treat this condition prior to injection. The usual treatment consists of lid hygiene and antibiotic drops or ointment. The clinician responsible will be able to guide you.

Regurgitation test. The lacrimal sac forms part of the lacrimal drainage system of the eyelids. This drains tears from openings in the inner aspect of the eyelids (called the puncta) down into the nose. An obstruction along this system can cause tears to collect in the lacrimal sac with subsequent infection. In the regurgitation test, the lacrimal sac is pressed with a finger (Fig. A.2) whilst the upper and lower puncta are observed with a slit lamp. Regurgitation through the puncta of yellow pus indicates infection and thus a higher chance of endophthalmitis after an intravitreal injection. This must be treated first by a responsible clinician. Treatment will normally include antibiotics to treat infection, with subsequent measures to try to resolve the obstruction (usually via a surgical procedure called a dacryocystorhinostomy).

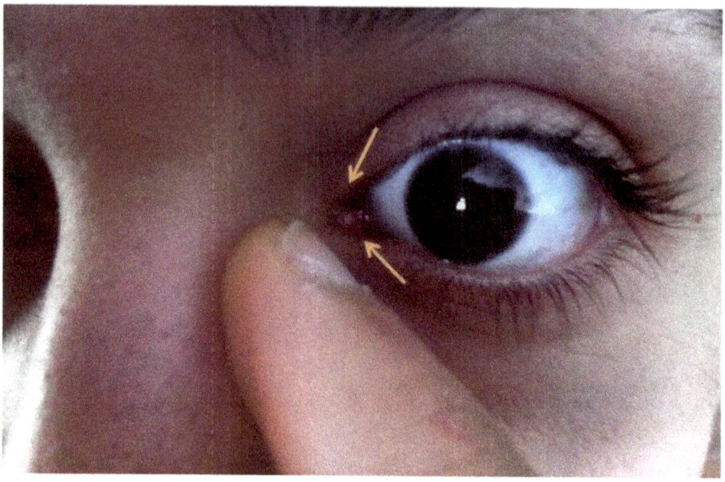

Fig. A.2. Regurgitation test: Press on the lacrimal sac with your finger as shown whilst observing the location of the puncta (arrows) for regurgitation.

APPENDIX B: BASIC LIFE SUPPORT ALGORITHM (RESUSCITATION COUNCIL, UK, 2015)

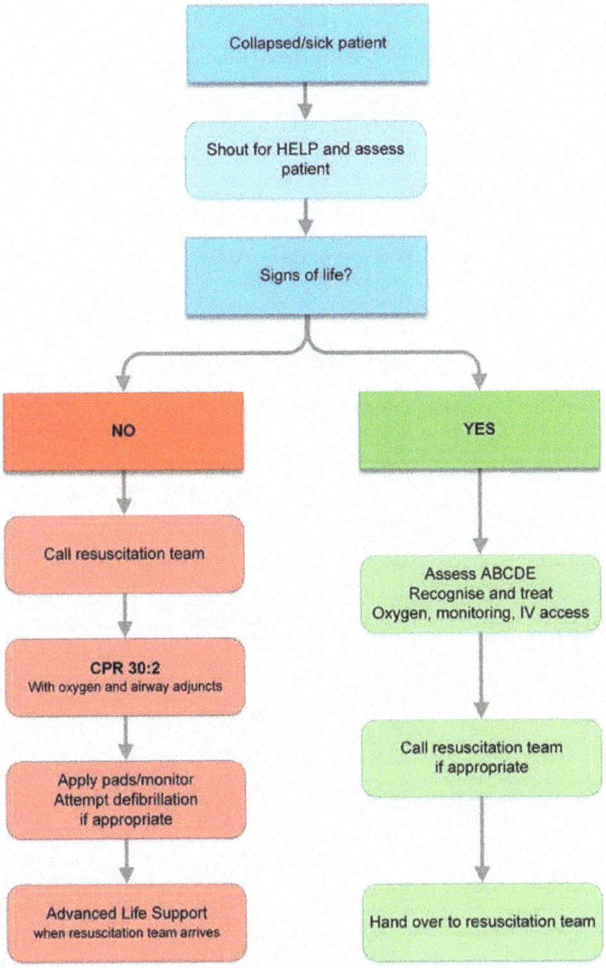

APPENDIX C: ANAPHYLAXIS ALGORITHM

Resuscitation Council (UK)

Anaphylaxis algorithm

Anaphylactic reaction?

↓

Airway, Breathing, Circulation, Disability, Exposure

↓

Diagnosis - look for:

- Acute onset of illness
- Life-threatening Airway and/or Breathing and/or Circulation problems [1]
- And usually skin changes

↓

- **Call for help**
- Lay patient flat
- Raise patient's legs

↓

Adrenaline [2]

↓

When skills and equipment available:

- Establish airway
- High flow oxygen
- IV fluid challenge [3]
- Chlorphenamine [4]
- Hydrocortisone [5]

Monitor:

- Pulse oximetry
- ECG
- Blood pressure

---

1 Life-threatening problems:

Airway:	swelling, hoarseness, stridor
Breathing:	rapid breathing, wheeze, fatigue, cyanosis, $SpO_2 < 92\%$, confusion
Circulation:	pale, clammy, low blood pressure, faintness, drowsy/coma

2 Adrenaline *(give IM unless experienced with IV adrenaline)*

IM doses of 1:1000 adrenaline (repeat after 5 min if no better)

• Adult	500 micrograms IM (0.5 mL)
• Child more than 12 years:	500 micrograms IM (0.5 mL)
• Child 6 -12 years:	300 micrograms IM (0.3 mL)
• Child less than 6 years:	150 micrograms IM (0.15 mL)

Adrenaline IV to be given **only by experienced specialists**
Titrate: Adults 50 micrograms; Children 1 microgram/kg

3 IV fluid challenge:

Adult - 500 – 1000 mL
Child - crystalloid 20 mL/kg

Stop IV colloid if this might be the cause of anaphylaxis

	4 Chlorphenamine (IM or slow IV)	**5 Hydrocortisone** (IM or slow IV)
Adult or child more than 12 years	10 mg	200 mg
Child 6 - 12 years	5 mg	100 mg
Child 6 months to 6 years	2.5 mg	50 mg
Child less than 6 months	250 micrograms/kg	25 mg

INDEX

www.ingramcontent.com/pod-product-compliance
Ingram Content Group UK Ltd.
Pitfield, Milton Keynes, MK11 3LW, UK
UKHW021531050225
4464UKWH00028B/353

9 789811 221323